Resveratrol - Recent Advances, Application, and Therapeutic Potential

Edited by Ali Imran and Hafiz A.R. Suleria

Published in London, United Kingdom

Resveratrol - Recent Advances, Application, and Therapeutic Potential
http://dx.doi.org/10.5772/intechopen.105313
Edited by Ali Imran and Hafiz A.R. Suleria

Contributors
Aftab Ahmed, Ali Imran, Ana Casas, Ana Novo Barros, Fakhar Islam, Farhan Saeed, Fatima Tariq, Ghulam Hussain, Hafiz A.R. Suleria, Javier Fidalgo, Jia-Ping Wu, Li Xiaoqing, Muhammad Afzaal, Muhammad Armghan Khalid, Muhammad Sadiq Naseer, Muhammad Umair Arshad, Muhammad Usama, Nosheen Amjad, Osman Tuncay Agar, Qasim Ali, Rabia Akram, Rabia Shabir Ahmad, Rehman Ali, Sadaf Khurshid, Umber Shehzadi, Usman Naeem, Veronique Traynard, Zhang Jie, Zhang Qian-Cheng, Zhu Xiaoning

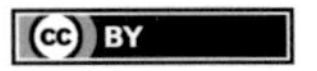

First published in London, United Kingdom, 2024 by IntechOpen
IntechOpen is the global imprint of INTECHOPEN LIMITED, registered in England and Wales, registration number: 11086078, 167-169 Great Portland Street, London, W1W 5PF, United Kingdom

British Library Cataloguing-in-Publication Data
A catalogue record for this book is available from the British Library

Additional hard and PDF copies can be obtained from orders@intechopen.com

Resveratrol - Recent Advances, Application, and Therapeutic Potential
Edited by Ali Imran and Hafiz A.R. Suleria
p. cm.
Print ISBN 978-1-83768-152-5
Online ISBN 978-1-83768-153-2
eBook (PDF) ISBN 978-1-83768-154-9

For EU product safety concerns:
IN TECH d.o.o., Prolaz Marije Krucifikse Kozulić 3, 51000 Rijeka, Croatia,
info@intechopen.com or visit our website at intechopen.com.

Meet the editors

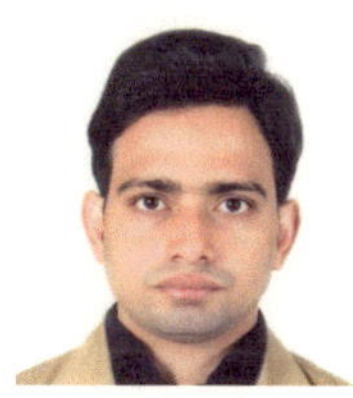

Dr. Ali Imran has been an associate professor in the Department of Food Sciences, Government College University, Faisalabad, Pakistan since 2013. He is an expert on polyphenol extraction, structural elucidation, and intervention preparation. He completed his postdoc at the University of Melbourne, Australia. His research focuses on the formulation of cost-effective polyphenol-based dietary interventions against various metabolic syndromes. He has mentored more than 30 graduate students and published more than 120 research articles. He has given more than fifty invited/keynote presentations throughout the world. Dr. Imran has served as scientific editor of two international journals.

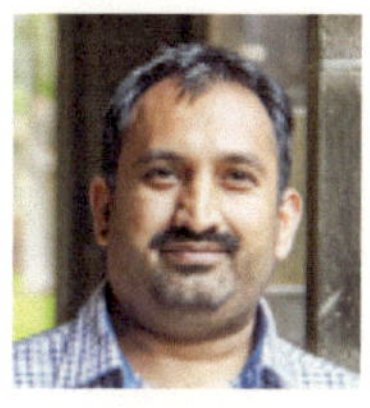

Hafiz A.R. Suleria is a senior lecturer (ARC DECRA Fellow) in the School of Agriculture and Food, University of Melbourne (UoM), Australia. Prior to the ARC DECRA Fellowship, he completed a McKenzie Fellowship (UoM), Alfred Deakin Fellowship (Deakin University, Australia), and US Postdoctoral Fellowship (Kansas State University, USA) in the field of food science and nutrition. Dr. Suleria's research focuses on food science and nutrition, particularly the screening of phytochemicals and bioactive molecules from different plant, marine, and animal sources. He has published more than 200 peer-reviewed scientific papers in journals. He also collaborates with more than five universities as a co-supervisor/special member for Ph.D. students and works on joint publications, projects, and grants.

Contents

Preface

This book, *Resveratrol – Recent Advances, Application, and Therapeutic Potential*, explores the promising therapeutic use of resveratrol antioxidants for lifestyle-related ailments. It covers a wide range of subjects, including significant studies on naturally occurring abundant phytochemicals in resveratrol. The book is a useful tool for postgraduate students and pharmaceutical professionals looking for current and crucially significant information on natural products.

The book contains five chapters written by leading researchers. After the introductory chapter, the book discusses the molecular processes of resveratrol involved in disease management. Then, it examines the chemistry, physicochemical characteristics, and chemical properties of resveratrol. The last two chapters deal with the therapeutic potential of this antioxidant with specific molecular targets.

This book is a must-read for anyone who wishes to learn more about the causes and available treatments for lifestyle-related ailments, including doctors, nutritionists, and scientists who study food and nutrition.

I hope the evaluations contained herein prove insightful and helpful to readers and encourage more research in the hunt for cutting-edge treatments for a variety of conditions. I wish to express my gratitude to the staff at IntechOpen for their valuable assistance.

Ali Imran
Department of Food Science,
Government College University,
Faisalabad, Pakistan

School of Agriculture, Food and Ecosystem Sciences,
Faculty of Science,
The University of Melbourne,
Parkville, VIC, Australia

Hafiz A.R. Suleria
School of Agriculture, Food and Ecosystem Sciences,
Faculty of Science,
The University of Melbourne,
Parkville, VIC, Australia

Section 1

Introduction

Chapter 1

Introductory Chapter: Resveratrol – Recent Advances, Application, and Therapeutic Potential

Nosheen Amjad, Fakhar Islam, Muhammad Usama, Qasim Ali, Muhammad Armghan Khalid, Usman Naeem, Muhammad Umair Arshad, Osman Tuncay Agar, Hafiz A.R. Suleria and Ali Imran

1. Introduction

Owing to its conceivable health advantages, resveratrol has received a great deal of interest lately. One such is the "French paradox," where despite the French population's excessive consumption of saturated fat, red wine drinking, which has a high resveratrol concentration, has been related to reduced cardiovascular disease mortality in the population. Since then, resveratrol has been the subject of extensive research aimed at a range of diverse health-beneficial impacts, which include however are not restricted to those related to anti-obesity, anti-inflammation, cardiovascular protection, antidiabetes type 2, anti-aging, anti-carcinogenesis, and neuroprotection [1]. Resveratrol has undergone significant research on a wide range of illnesses, but it has also been tested for its ability to fight against germs and fungi. The stilbene family of naturally stirring polyphenolic antioxidants includes resveratrol (3,5,4′-trihydroxystilbene). Resveratrol is a hydroxylated derivative of a stilbene with a C6-C2-C6 carbon skeleton (1,2- diphenylethylene). Numerous plants, including grapevines (*Vitis vinifera*), blueberries, cranberries (Vaccinium spp.), and peanuts (Arachis hypogea), as well as traditional Asian herbal medicines, contain resveratrol. However, grapevines are the primary natural source for human consumption. Resveratrol is a naturally up phytoalexin that a plant produces when they are damaged by fungus or ultraviolet (UV) rays [2]. As evidenced by the Botrytis cinerea fungus, the cause of gray mold. According to Jeandet et al. [3], the production of resveratrol is more common in the grapes that are not infected but are in close proximity to grapevines that have been infected with a fungus. This mechanism helps in inhibiting the spread of infection to the healthy grapes. Both a cis and a trans isomer of resveratrol exist; the opposite geometric isomer is the supplementary predominant arrangement in red wine and is the subject of the utmost research because of its higher bioavailability and increased stability. Overall, red wine has more resveratrol than white wine. Trans-resveratrol levels in red wine can range from 1.9 mg/L on average to 14.3 mg/L,

IntechOpen

according to Stervbo et al. [4]. Over twenty proteins in eukaryotic species interact with the promiscuous chemical resveratrol. Resveratrol has the ability to attach itself to the F1-domain of bovine ATP synthase, specifically within a small space located between a β-subunit and the γ-subunit, as demonstrated by crystallization complexes [5]. The maintenance of the Mitochondrial ATPase or ATP synthase residues implies that *Escherichia coli* has a comparable binding site for resveratrol. In *E. coli*, a facultative aerobe, resveratrol has the ability to bind to ATP synthase in a reversible manner. This binding process leads to a partial obstruction of both ATP hydrolysis and synthesis.

2. Therapeutic application

Resveratrol lowers the metabolic rate of *Arcobacter spp.* and inhibits *Mycobacterium smegmatis*'s hydrolysis of Adenosine triphosphate. Resveratrol administration to *E. coli* chambers decreases the growth of fermentable glucose and prohibits development of the non-fermentable source of carbon succinate, which indicates that resveratrol suppresses oxidative phosphorylation. According to Boogerd et al. [6], the growth of *E. coli* mutants lacking ATP synthase can still occur in the presence of fermentable carbon sources such as glucose, pyruvate, or lactate. This suggests that ATP synthase alone cannot be the sole target responsible for inhibiting growth in *E. coli*. Furthermore, in *E. coli*, resveratrol induces DNA fragmentation and leads to the upregulation of the SOS stress-response regulon. Yet, growth suppression is not a direct result of DNA fragmentation or the elevation of the SOS stress response. The cellular multiplication machinery is also impacted by resveratrol due to the elongation of resveratrol-treated *E. coli* cells, which happens when ftsZ expression is suppressed. Resveratrol is considered to obstruct FtsZ-mediated septum formation and cellular replication since FtsZ is a crucial protein in septum synthesis throughout cellular replication. Subramanian et al. [7] found that resveratrol administration was associated with cell membrane damage because it enhanced potassium leakage and propidium iodide absorption. Whereas *Staphylococcus aureus* Nohr-Meldgaard et al. [8] found no evidence of resveratrol-induced membrane damage. Numerous human investigations have shown that after oral administration, resveratrol exhibits significant absorption but limited bioavailability of unaltered resveratrol. Following oral treatment, resveratrol is easily metabolized; sulfate- and glucuronide-resveratrol conjugates achieve plasma concentrations that are 3–8 times greater than those of free resveratrol. Following a single oral dose of 5 g of trans-resveratrol, the peak plasma concentration of resveratrol reached 539 ng/mL after 1.5 hours. However, the average plasma concentration decreased to approximately 52 ng/mL after 24 hours. Similarly, to this, after taking 1 g of resveratrol orally, the average plasma concentration was 73 ng/mL. Given the inhibitory doses required, the systemic application of resveratrol for the treatment of infections caused by bacteria is restricted by the limited bioavailability of orally given resveratrol. It could be intriguing to look into the antibacterial qualities of such conjugates given that in humans, resveratrol undergoes rapid metabolism, resulting in higher levels of resveratrol conjugates in the bloodstream compared to the unmodified form of the molecule. The effects of resveratrol administered intravenously (IV) in humans have also been studied, but the directed dosage was small, being 0.2 mg, and it was rapidly metabolized, suggesting that i.v. resveratrol administration might have limited, if any, anti-microbial uses for systemic diseases. Furthermore, the application of resveratrol topically offers the potential to utilize concentrations that have a beneficial effect against numerous infectious diseases, as suggested by Zhou et al. [9].

3. Conclusion

In the nutshell, the resveratrol holds medicinal and preservative activity mainly attributed to its strong antioxidant potential. Moreover, it showed the tendency to be used in the formulation of different functional products. Furthermore, more human-based efficacy trials are suggested to unveil its true therapeutic potential.

Author details

Nosheen Amjad[1], Fakhar Islam[1,2], Muhammad Usama[2], Qasim Ali[3], Muhammad Armghan Khalid[2], Usman Naeem[4], Muhammad Umair Arshad[2], Osman Tuncay Agar[5], Hafiz A.R. Suleria[5] and Ali Imran[2,5]*

1 Department of Clinical Nutrition, NUR International University, Lahore, Pakistan

2 Department of Food Science, Government College University, Faisalabad, Pakistan

3 Department of Botany, Government College University, Faisalabad, Pakistan

4 Faculty of Diet and Nutritional Sciences, Department of Diet and Nutritional Sciences, University of Lahore, Lahore, Pakistan

5 School of Agriculture, Food and Ecosystem Sciences, Faculty of Science, The University of Melbourne, Parkville VIC, Australia

*Address all correspondence to: dr.aliimran@gcuf.edu.pk

References

[1] Timmers S, Hesselink MK, Schrauwen P. Therapeutic potential of resveratrol in obesity and type 2 diabetes: New avenues for health benefits? Annals of the New York Academy of Sciences. 2013;**1290**(1):83-89

[2] Langcake P, Pryce RJ. The production of resveratrol by Vitis vinifera and other members of the Vitaceae as a response to infection or injury. Physiological Plant Pathology. 1976;**9**(1):77-86

[3] Jeandet P, Bessis R, Sbaghi M, Meunier P. Production of the phytoalexin resveratrol by grapes as a response to Botrytis attack under natural conditions. Journal of Phytopathology. 1995;**143**(3):135-139

[4] Stervbo U, Vang O, Bonnesen C. A review of the content of the putative chemopreventive phytoalexin resveratrol in red wine. Food Chemistry. 2007;**101**(2):449-457

[5] Gledhill JR, Montgomery MG, Leslie AG, Walker JE. Mechanism of inhibition of bovine F1-ATPase by resveratrol and related polyphenols. Proceedings of the National Academy of Sciences. 2007;**104**(34):13632-13637

[6] Boogerd FC, Boe L, Michelsen OLE, Jensen PR. ATP mutants of Escherichia coli fail to grow on succinate due to a transport deficiency. Journal of Bacteriology. 1998;**180**(22):5855-5859

[7] Subramanian M, Goswami M, Chakraborty S, Jawali N. Resveratrol induced inhibition of Escherichia coli proceeds via membrane oxidation and independent of diffusible reactive oxygen species generation. Redox Biology. 2014;**2**:865-872

[8] Nøhr-Meldgaard K, Ovsepian A, Ingmer H, Vestergaard M. Resveratrol enhances the efficacy of aminoglycosides against *Staphylococcus aureus*. International Journal of Antimicrobial Agents. 2018;**52**(3):390-396

[9] Zhou JW, Chen TT, Tan XJ, Sheng JY, Jia AQ. Can the quorum sensing inhibitor resveratrol function as an aminoglycoside antibiotic accelerant against *Pseudomonas aeruginosa*? International Journal of Antimicrobial Agents. 2018;**52**(1):35-41

Section 2

Phytochemistry: Resveratrol

Chapter 2

Resveratrol Synthesis, Metabolism, and Delivery: A Mechanistic Treatise

Fakhar Islam, Umber Shehzadi, Farhan Saeed, Rabia Shabir Ahmad, Muhammad Umair Arshad, Muhammad Sadiq Naseer, Fatima Tariq, Rehman Ali, Sadaf Khurshid, Ghulam Hussain, Aftab Ahmad, Muhammad Afzaal, Rabia Akram, Osman Tuncay Agar, Ali Imran and Hafiz A.R. Suleria

Abstract

Resveratrol, a bioactive phytochemical classified as a phytoalexin present in plant sources, is recognized for its distinct characteristics such as anticancer, chemoprotective, chemosensitizer, neuroprotective, anti-inflammatory, and antioxidant properties. Resveratrol is a polyphenol that increases the susceptibility of cancer-resistant cells to chemotherapy. Resveratrol also aids in weight loss by decreasing lipogenesis, the prevention of neurological illnesses, and other topical uses such as the treatment of skin hyperpigmentation. During the past 10 years, resveratrol, a naturally occurring stilbene found in various foods and drinks, has drawn increased interest due to its many health benefits, including its chemo-preventive and anticancer actions. Several naturally occurring resveratrol derivatives can be found in food and share a similar structural makeup with resveratrol. To boost the effectiveness and activity of particular resveratrol features, several resveratrol analogues have also been created by the addition of designated functional groups. Such resveratrol derivatives might provide beneficial cancer therapeutics and cancer chemo-preventive drugs for cancer prevention and therapy. However, the quest for the identification of new analogues with high yield must be explored to extend resveratrol effectiveness. This chapter provides an overview of the most significant resveratrol derivatives used to treat cardiovascular diseases and the methods of their synthesis.

Keywords: resveratrol, therapeutic potential, antioxidants, phytochemicals, metabolism

1. Introduction

As a consequence of breakthroughs in nutritional research, academics have shown that nutrition plays a vital role in a number of disorders. Many investigations into the molecular effects of phytoconstituents have demonstrated that they are both safe and effective for long-term treatment. Recently, it has been found that several phytochemicals have strong anticancer and anti-arthritic properties. They consist of tea polyphenols, rosmarinic acid, curcumin, and resveratrol [1]. Polyphenol resveratrol may be found in a wide variety of plants [2]. It has cis and trans configurations, which can occasionally change toward one-up difference because a C=C double bond is present. White squash was where resveratrol was first discovered in the 1940s; since then, it has also been discovered in grapes, peanuts, and *Polygonum cuspidatum*, among other plants [3].

Because of its abundance, and significant health advantages following ingestion, merlot, a biologically active polyphenolic stilbenoid, has gained interest in the management of medical conditions [4]. Research has been done on this molecule's antioxidant, anti-inflammatory, and anti-carcinogenic characteristics, and most relate to lowering oxidative stress. Moreover, it has been shown to mediate autophagy, govern critical homeostatic processes in the body, and provide a range of systemic protective advantages [5].

Conventional β-cell cancer treatments including chemotherapy, surgery, and radiation have a number of drawbacks, including the ability to destroy healthy tissue and toxicity and long-term repercussions. Production of bioactives like resveratrol has been suggested as a feasible method of therapy to address these problems [6]. The use of nanoformulations in cancer treatment has been expanded upon to provide targeted distribution and improve valuable benefits. As compared to the way these drugs are typically administered, the use of nanoformulations of biotherapeutics has been shown to boost therapeutic value by increasing absorption and, ultimately, permeability. One such significant advance is the application of immunology [7]. Chimeric antigen receptor (CAR)-T β-cell lymphomas that are malignant have been treated using immunotherapy. Second-generation anti-CD19 medicines have gained prompt regulatory clearance and have been the subject of in-depth study in the treatment of relapse patients. Nevertheless, a few delivery and toxicity-related problems need to be overcome before they may be used more generally [8]. To solve the shortcomings of traditional drug delivery methods, this research focuses on the synthesis of resveratrol and describes the evidence for the related molecular mechanisms underlying these effects. This chapter also discusses the positive advantages of resveratrol, as well as the many hurdles connected with resveratrol's clinical development and future prospects for therapeutic uses of this agent.

2. Synthesis and derivatives of resveratrol

With researchers' discovery of organic merlot, several attempts have been undertaken to chemically and biologically develop resveratrol.

2.1 Heck reaction

The C−C coupling of an engaged olefin with an aryl or vinyl halide is known as the Heck reaction, which is accelerated by palladium in the presence of a base. There are many acceptors and donors that are acceptable for Heck interactions, owing to subsequent advancements in catalytic and heterogeneous catalysts. Resveratrol and its substitutes can only be produced by the Forget interaction [9].

Pd catalysts from various sources must be immobilized onto heterogeneous supports to create pterostilbene. In addition to studying the structure of resveratrol derivatives, important polyphenolic compounds may be synthesized via retrosynthesis methods [10]. Palladium nanoparticles supported on synthetic clay may be able to successfully drive the Heck-Mizoroki C—C cross-coupling reaction, an essential step. This reaction's catalyst is strong, stable, and controlled. A tiny number of solvents is required during the purifying process, and the catalyst may be recovered and reused numerous times. Via a decarbonylative Heck process, the phytoalexin resveratrol may be produced. By combining 3,5-dihydroxybenzoic acid and 4-acetoxystyrene with palladium acetate and N,N-bis-(2,6diisopropylphenyl) dihydroimidazolium chloride, resveratrol derivatives were produced during this process [11]. Scientists have successfully synthesized a variety of resveratrol mimics. In experiments on human HL-60 cells, the four-acetoxy derivatives of resveratrol showed enhanced activity (ED50). A study team developed a brand-new, 70% yielding, effective method for producing resveratrol. Researchers improved the synthesis procedures, resulting in a 22–71% increase in overall resveratrol yield [12].

Scientists could synthesize resveratrol in a method that was rapid, simple, and incredibly chemo-, regio-, and stereoselective by dividing the tannin structure into three parts. Some of these derivatives were successful at protecting thymocytes from radioactive material apoptosis, studying of the radioprotective capabilities of resveratrol derivatives. Researchers looked into the manufacturing when utilizing the same procedure but changing the ring structure to a phenol ring [13]. The components demonstrated strong anti-human breast cancer cell activity. Researchers used a number of *in vitro* and cell-based targets to synthesize resveratrol via the Heck reaction to compare its activity to that of sulphate metabolites. Metabolites of sulphate are frequently less powerful than merlot [14].

2.2 Perkin reaction

Spontaneously, the Perkin synthesis transforms aromatic aldehydes and anhydrides into alpha- and beta-unsaturated carboxylic acids. It requires sodium acetate, an acid, and a base. Phases of the process include condensation, decarboxylation, deprotection, and protection. A product of the regioselective reaction is developed. Späth and Kromp first produced resveratrol using the Perkin reaction, which calls for 1,3-dimethoxy benzaldehyde and sodium salt of p-anisyl acetic acid as the reactants in the presence of acetic anhydride. Takaoka started synthesizing resveratrol after finding it in the root plant Veratrum grandfluorum. The final resveratrol derivative product, which has a structure precisely like a natural substance, was created by decarboxylating quinolone-Cu salt. Many advancements have been noticed [15].

2.3 Wittig reaction

The Wittig reactions use triphenylphosphine, a base, and a byproduct termed triphenylphosphine-oxide to change the main primary alkyl halides, aldehydes/ketones, and an olefin output to make an olefin product. This technique typically resulted in a C=C double bond. By using the Wittig reaction, we produced trans-resveratrol and investigated how grapes produced resveratrol berries at various phases of growth. Resveratrol was either absent from or present in tiny amounts in the flesh of the fruit; it was generated in the skin cells. The amount of resveratrol in grape skin and the phases of berry development were clearly inversely correlated. If the phosphoric geographical region allies are benzyl alcohols, resveratrol and its analogues are synthesized in a single-pot Wittig-type olefination process. By using the Wittig reaction, we were able to produce trans-resveratrol [16].

Even though the Baeyer process is often employed to create an ethylenic bridge, it produces triphenylphosphine oxide as a byproduct and has poor trans invention yields and/or low E/Z selectivity. As a result, chromatography purifying is necessary for the procedure. Thus, it is crucial to look for rapid processing techniques or efficient catalysts for Wittig interactions [17].

2.4 Other methods

In addition to the typical resveratrol reactions, researchers have found additional ways to make resveratrol and its derivatives. Studies have compiled recent advancements in the Julia-Kocienski response, and the reaction has been recognized as a vital step in the synthesis of resveratrol [18]. The reactants were 3,5-dimethoxybenzyl trimethylsilyl ether and a number of aldehydes. Metallic lithium was created after a sequence of reactions, producing the required reaction result. Scientists have used a conventional Horner-Emmons-Wadsworth reaction or a Sonogashira-type reaction to manufacture resveratrol in huge quantities [13].

Using aluminum chloride induction, researchers recovered resveratrol from grapevine leaves. Also, using this technique, Botrytis cinerea in vineyards may be managed. Researchers have also developed methods for producing resveratrol and its analogues using biosynthesis and biomimicry. Researchers also transformed apples using *Agrobacterium tumefaciens*, and they found that this transformation can create resveratrol with stable inheritance [19]. Researchers have discovered that when synthesizing resveratrol and its equivalents by chemo-enzymatic reaction, the procedure delivers a sustained produce of the preceding produce. Fifty-seven other strategies have also been employed [20].

3. Resveratrol derivatives

As a result, several variants have been invented to boost this molecule's effectiveness and stability. There are several publications that go into great lengths about the results and uses of resveratrol derivatives. A brief summary of these substances is given in **Table 1**. By lowering ROS production and protecting oxidative phosphorylation capability, HS-1793 protected mitochondria from cardiac ischemia/reperfusion injury. These resveratrol compounds therefore have a high therapeutic promise for both CVD and a variety of cancers [28].

3.1 Absorption of resveratrol

Resveratrol is known to have the characteristics of low water solubility, which is reported to be <0.05 mg/mL owing to its chemical structure. Solubility of resveratrol can be enhanced by introducing organic solvents or alcoholic compounds [29]. The ability of resveratrol to form complexes organically with aliphatic hydrocarbons due to the presence of hydroxyl group is the pathway that can be opted for increasing intestinal absorption as well as permeability of cellular walls of enterocytes. It is also absorbed via passive diffusion and transferred in the circulatory system [30]. Free-form sulphate or glucuronide are the altered forms of resveratrol existing in human blood. Free resveratrol has shown low affinity to albumin, predicting that it is a naturally occurring polyphenol reservoir that can bind to human plasma lipoproteins and enter the cells via portal circulation (**Figure 1**) [31].

Nanoformulations	Chemical Composition	Observation	Reference
Resveratrol Microparticles	Usage of magnesium dihydorixde as a supporting base	Improvement of solubility and subsequently bioavailability	[21]
Resveratrol encapsulated with silica carrier	Encapsulation of the drug alongside functional silica carriers, matrix-type drug release	Maintenance of cytotoxic properties, improvement of solubility profile	[22]
Resveratrol nanoparticles	Loading of the drug onto a chitosan-pectin core	Provision of sustained drug delivery, improved activity, easy modulation of release by variation of parameters	[23]
Resveratrol + Gefitinib cocrystals	Combination of resveratrol with a synthetic chemotherapeutic agent	Improved stability as well as solubility, indicating potential for increased clinical usage	[24]
Nanocomplexation of resveratrol with nanofibrils	Fabricated pea protein isolate (PPI) nanofibrils+ resveratrol	Significantly improved solubility, greater surface area for drug incorporation, greater antioxidant potential even at low doses	[25]
Resveratrol loaded nanoparticles (NPs)	Chitosan and γ-poly(glutamic acid) (γ-PGA)	Improved UV stability and enhanced solubility and antioxidant property	[26]
Resveratrol loaded onto nanosponges	Combination of resveratrol and oxyresveratrol	Improved UV stability, solubility as well as antioxidant effect, as well as a satisfactory toxicity profile	[27]

Table 1.
Nanotechnological advancements in resveratrol delivery.

3.2 Metabolism of resveratrol

The metabolism of resveratrol has been studied and shown using a variety of experimental methodologies. It has been noticed that metabolic enzymes and gut bacteria are both necessary for its biotransformation. Moreover, the amount given, any ongoing medical problems, sex, and tissues all have an impact on the rate of metabolism [32].

Members of the UGT family of enzymes catalyze the conjugation of resveratrol with a glucuronic acid moiety at the 3 or 40 hydroxyl group position, changing the antioxidant's medicinal properties and accelerating its excretion from the body. Human liver microsomes (HLMs) have a large number of UGT enzymes, allowing them to produce more 3-O-glucuronide than 40-O-glucuronide preferentially. Sulfation is a further mechanism of metabolizing tannin. Human sulfotransferase may sulphate resveratrol to one of three different degrees, resulting in resveratrol-3-O-sulfate, resveratrol-40-Osulfate, and resveratrol-3, 40-O-disulfate, according to a study [33].

Moreover, research has demonstrated that resveratrol injection may be a viable therapy for lupus nephritis in MRL/lpr mice by increasing the activity of FcRIIB, allowing the selective removal of B-cells from the bone marrow and the spleen [34]. Resveratrol inhibits Stat3 at low doses, which inhibits the development and function

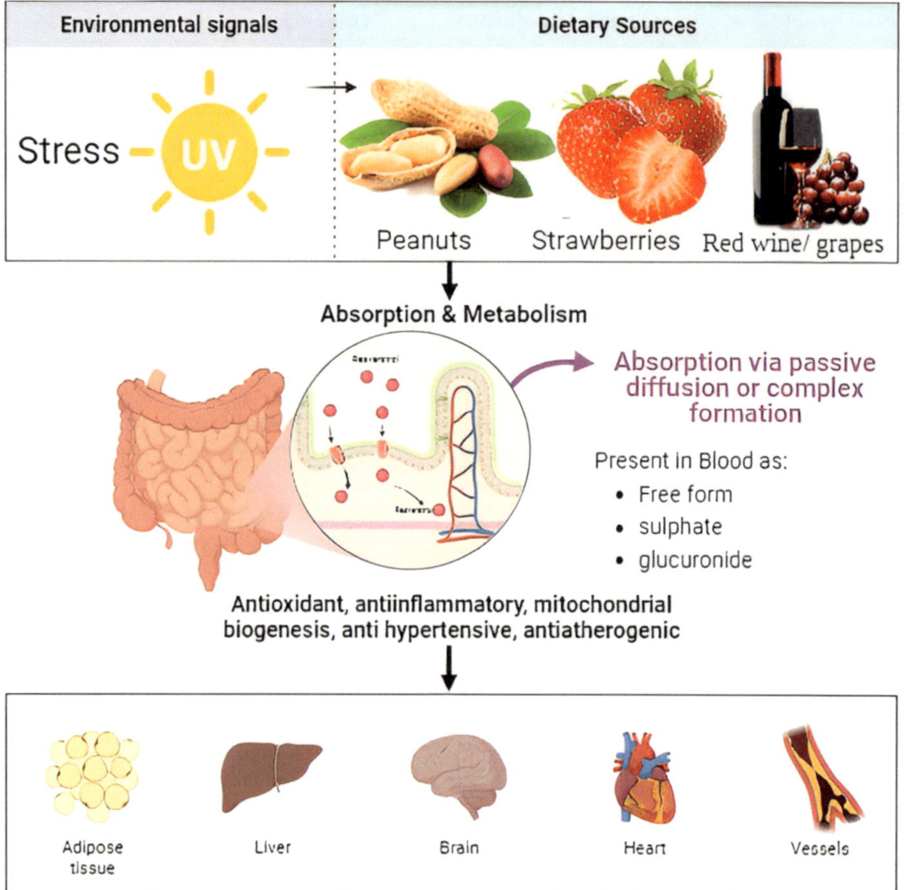

Figure 1.
Absorption of resveratrol.

of tumor-evoked regulatory B-cells. As TGF is a downstream target of Stat3, this prevents it from being able to express itself [35].

3.3 Nanotechnological interventions

Because of the poor bioavailability of resveratrol (said to be less than 0.05 mg/mL), dosage has been severely hampered. When mixing circumstances were ideal, the solubility of resveratrol in peanut oil achieved up to 95% [36]. Resveratrol was able to maintain its antioxidant action and extend its shelf life even in a lipid-based solvent. This suggested that peanut oil may be employed as a drug carrier during the formulation design phase as illustrated in **Table 2** [40].

The solubility and stability of this phytochemical have been attempted to be increased using a variety of nanotechnological treatments. To extend the time that the drug remains in the body and, as a result, boost bioavailability, many nanoformulations have been utilized [41]. In addition to these benefits, using nanoformulations significantly lessens medication metabolism, principally by decreasing glucuronidation. To enhance the dispersion of this drug and reduce problems with its stability and absorption, nanotechnological interventions present a considerable possibility [42].

Derivatives		Applications	Effects	References
Hydroxylated resveratrol derivatives	Dihydroxystilbene	Anticancer	Antiagiogenic effect, inhibits migration	[37]
	Tetramethoxystilbene	Anticancer,	Antioxidative effect, antiangiogenic effect	[28]
	trimethoxy-benzamidine	hypertension	Inhibits DNA synthesis	[38]
Other resveratrol derivatives	Mitochondria-targeted resveratrol derivatives	Anticancer, mitochondrial regulation	Enhance solubility, mitochondria targeting	[39]
	Pterostilbene	Anticancer	Enhances bioavailability, antioxidative eff	[37]
	Hexahydroxystilbene	Anticancer	NF-KB inhibition, SOD inhibition	[28]
Methoxylated resveratrol derivatives	Tetrahydroxystilbene	Ischemic heart disease	Apoptosis regulation, KATP channel opening	
	Resveratrol triacetate	Anticancer	Cell cycle arrest	[39]
	Fluorinated stilbenes	Anticancer	Antiproliferative effect	[37]
	Digalloylresveratrol	Anticancer	Apoptosis regulation	[38]

Table 2.
Resveratrol derivatives effects therapeutically.

4. Resveratrol role in cardiovascular disease

4.1 Antiatherogenic effects of resveratrol

The primary mechanism behind the early onset of atherosclerotic lesions is the transformation of macrophages into foam cells following an excessive ingestion of lipoprotein. It's noteworthy to notice that resveratrol affects a number of chemical agents involved in the lipid metabolism of macrophages (**Figure 2**) [43].

Prostaglandin E2, a significant inflammatory substance, is produced by COX-2 (PGE2). Resveratrol controls COX-2 transcriptional activity, preventing PGE2 generation and limiting the inflammatory response to atherosclerosis. PPAR-c, which also has antiatherogenic effects on smooth muscle cells, endothelial cells, and macrophages, promotes modified low-density lipoprotein (LDL) uptake and macrophage maturation. Hence, PPAR-c agonists may have anti-inflammatory properties that help with atherosclerosis prevention. The LXR activation that resveratrol induces must regulate the atherogenesis process [44]. Transmembrane proteins called ABC transporters hydrolyze ATP, and the energy released makes it easier for molecules to cross cell membranes. The inflammatory cardiovascular aberrations associated with aging have recently been related to resveratrol supplementation [45].

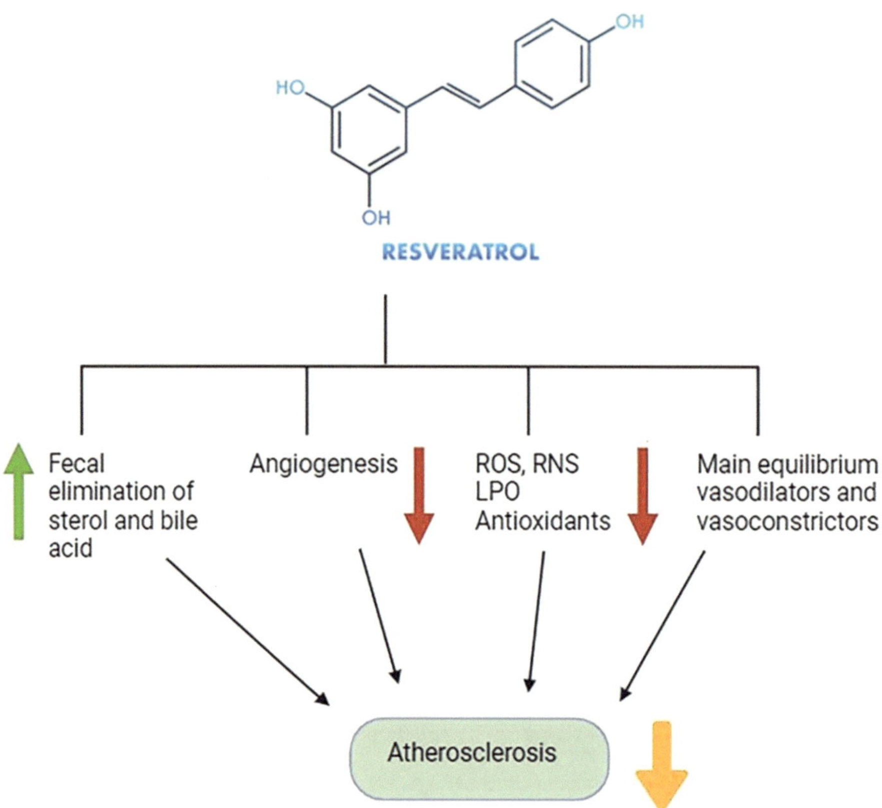

Figure 2.
Antiatherogenic effects of RES.

4.2 Anti-inflammatory effects of resveratrol

The relevance of developmental vicissitudes in addition to the outmoded jeopardy influences for the growth of CVD is highlighted by recent research. For example, in elderly persons, inferior irritation related with aging raises the risk of coronary artery infection and stroke. Many studies lend credence to the hypothesis that augmented NAD(P)H oxidase action and excessive mitochondrial reactive oxygen species (ROS) formation cause inflammation and endothelial damage as well as the vascular oxidative stress associated with aging [46].

NO, which is essential for preserving endothelial cell activity, seems to be a key ingredient in developmental vicissitudes. NO becomes inactive due to high superoxide concentrations brought on by oxidative damage brought on by aging. Vasomotor dysfunction is severe, endothelial cell death is elevated, and mitochondrial biogenesis is compromised as a result [47].

Recently, resveratrol supplementation has been recommended as a means of preventing the proatherogenic vascular vicissitudes connected to maturing. Resveratrol increases eNOS expression and enhances NO bioavailability, both of which are consistent with these potential benefits. By correcting the physiological changes brought on by oxidative stress and aging, resveratrol acts as a vasoprotective in animals. Moreover, resveratrol inhibits vascular NADPH oxidases, downregulates

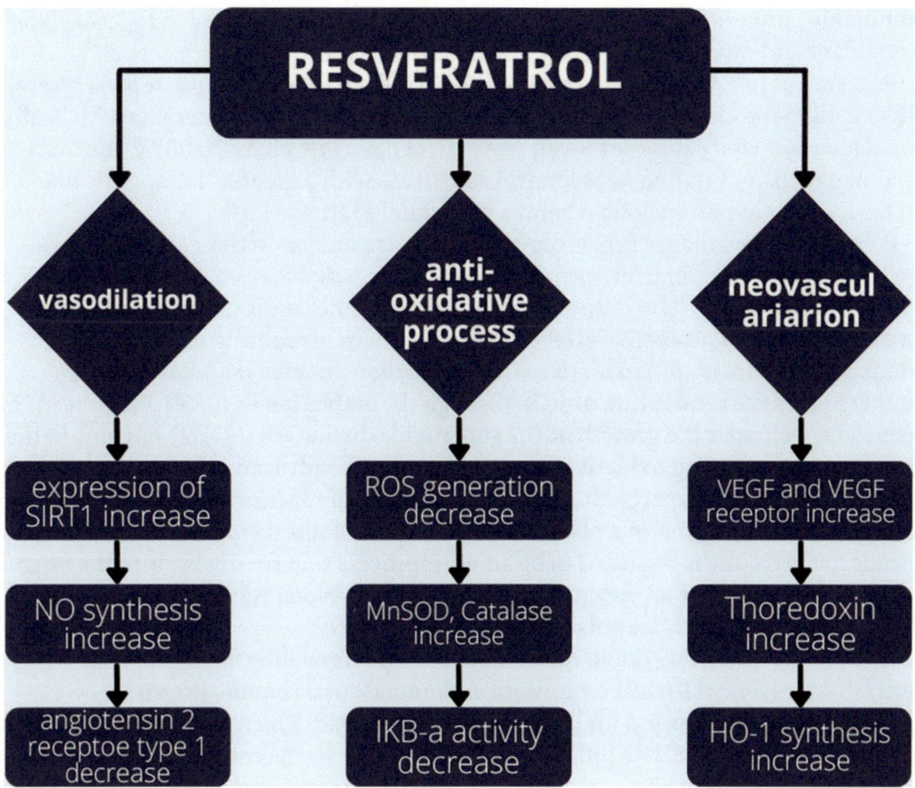

Figure 3.
The antihypertensive effects of resveratrol.

the expression of tumor necrosis factor-a in vascular and cardiac tissues, and may also prevent the production of mitochondrial ROS in the vascular system (**Figure 3**) [48].

4.3 Antihypertensive effects of resveratrol

The defining characteristic of the medical condition hypertension is a rise in arterial blood pressure over time. Almost one-fourth of people globally have hypertension. This therapeutic complaint raises the jeopardy of peripheral ischemic heart attack, vascular infection, and stroke, making it possibly the most significant and treatable risk factor for early mortality worldwide. According to the current study, resveratrol may reduce blood pressure through complex processes involving vasodilation, antioxidative activity, and neovascularization. Resveratrol targets sirtuins, and SIRT 1 is the sirtuin that has garnered the most attention from scientists [49].

The vascular endothelium generates more NO when resveratrol increases SIRT 1 expression, which results in vasodilation. Increased endothelial NO stimulates the production of hemeoxygenase-1 (HO-1), a precursor of bilirubin that also has antihypertensive properties. An endogenous vasopressor is ET-1 [50]. The cascading repercussions are examined, potentially linking the benefits of resveratrol in antiatherogenicity and increased longevity to the renin-angiotensin system [19, 51].

By preventing the generation of reactive oxygen species (ROS), phosphorylating Akt and p38 MAPK, activating IKB-α and NF-KB, and limiting the production of ROS, zinfandel safeguards the function of endothelial cells in the vascular system.

Tannins also promote the production of thioredoxin and HO-1, which together have antioxidant and myocardial angiogenesis properties [50].

Resveratrol functions better as a prophylactic drug than a treatment for irreversible vascular remodeling, based on our understanding of how it interacts with healthy vascular endothelial cells. Moreover, resveratrol has a low bioavailability due to its rapid metabolism. Finding a resveratrol substitute with a greater therapeutic potential for treating hypertension is therefore essential [52].

Polyphenol advantages for cardio-protection are unique to the significant positive belongings of resveratrol, even if these advantages have been demonstrated by several current researchers in spontaneous models of heart disease. Animal studies have confirmed the protective effects of resveratrol in preventing cardiac fibrosis, autophagy, apoptosis, and oxidative stress in cardiomyocytes [53]. Resveratrol notably lowers the production of ROS through the activation of SIRT1. Moreover, this chemical encourages the growth of the superoxide dismutase (SOD2) enzyme in the mitochondria, reducing oxidative stress in the mitochondria and the resulting cellular damage. Myocardial hypertrophic is the heart's natural reaction to hemodynamic tension brought on by numerous physiological and pathological conditions. Nonetheless, chronic hypertrophy is regarded to be an unfit process that finally leads to the organism's demise because of an elevated effort. There are several ways to explain how resveratrol prevents cardiac enlargement (**Table 3**) [59].

Resveratrol first slows down the obedience and remodeling of slight veins. In contrast, in resveratrol-treated rats with abdominal aortic bands, pressures overwhelm cardiac hypertrophy, and dysfunction is restored. The reason for these effects may be the rise in eNOS/NO [60]. The resveratrol blocks the serine-threonine kinase AMP-activated protein kinase (LKB1), a downstream signaling molecule, from being inhibited by oxidative stress (AMPK). Last but not least, resveratrol suppresses cardiac transcription of the angiotensin II receptor, AT1a, which helps to stop the development of heart hypertrophy [61].

Resveratrol has also been demonstrated to offer cardioprotective advantages in various situations. Since it results in cardiac enlargement and functional impairment, low ambient temperature is recognized as a substantial CVD jeopardy influence. Treatment with

Study Type	Dose and Time Period	Results	References
RCT	400 mg daily for 30 days	RES dramatically reduced the levels of VCAM, ICAM, and IL-8. In those with minimal cardiovascular risk, RES may have preventive benefits against the development of atherosclerosis.	Zhao et al. [54]
Meta-analysis	> 300 mg daily	Systolic blood pressure was considerably lowered with RES.	Fogacci et al. [55]
Meta-analysis	> 150 mg daily	RES dramatically lowered the amount of systolic blood pressure.	Liu et al. [56]
RCT	single dose (300 mg)	Women's FMD was considerably elevated by RES upon acute supplementation.	Marques et al. [57]
RCT	500 mg daily for 4 weeks	The levels of HDL cholesterol, the ratio of total to HDL cholesterol, and glycemic control were all improved by RES.	Hoseini et al. [58]

Table 3.
Cardio protective effects of RES.

resveratrol successfully inhibits these changes by preventing cardiomyocyte apoptosis [62]. Despite the common occurrence of autophagic dysfunction in diabetics, resveratrol promotes the growth of functional autophagy mechanisms within cells, has a positive impact on this diabetic cardiomyopathy. By preventing the ROS/ERK/TGF-b/periostin pathway from being activated, resveratrol reduces myocardium fibrosis in diabetic mice. Resveratrol also enhances the miR-130a gene, suppresses the miR-34a gene, blocks the miR-34a/Sirt1 gene, lowers oxidative stress, and lowers cardiac fibrosis and inflammation to protect against myocardial traumas brought on by myocardial infarction or hypoxia/reoxygenation damage [63].

As already noted, resveratrol defends the heart from endogenous causes like irritation, dyslipidemia, and endothelial dysfunction. Whether resveratrol also shields the myocardium from external elements like therapeutic medicines or endotoxin lipopolysaccharides has been the subject of more recent studies. Moreover, doxorubicin's anticancer effects are enhanced by resveratrol by increasing its cellular absorption. These results suggest that resveratrol might reduce cardiotoxicity and work in concert with doxorubicin to kill cancer cells (**Figure 4**) [64].

4.4 Antimetabolic syndrome

The metabolic condition is a lingering criticism that increases the jeopardy of diabetes and cardiovascular syndrome. This disease is characterized by the occurrence of, at the slightest, three of the subsequent health issues: elevated fasting glucose, high blood pressure, high serum triglycerides, high blood sugar, and abdominal (central) obesity. Metabolic syndrome, which affects around one-fourth of adult populations globally, is rather common in modern civilizations [65]. Nowadays, drugs to treat hypercholesterolemia are used as part of the treatment for metabolic syndrome. Insulin performs to be the primary hormone implicated in metabolic syndrome,

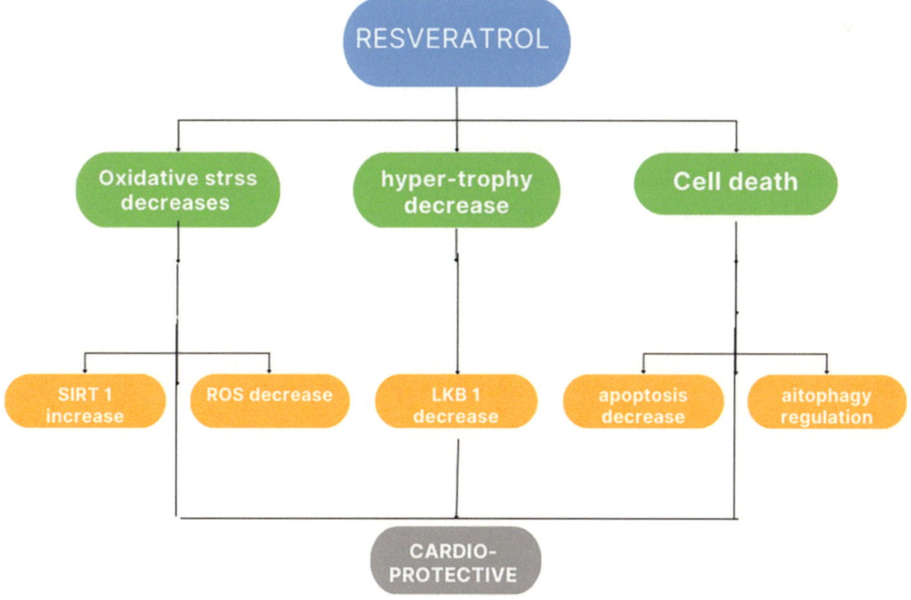

Figure 4.
Illustration of the cardioprotective effects of resveratrol.

despite the datum that the pathophysiology of this disorder is incredibly complicated and only slightly altered. According to some professionals, prediabetes and metabolic syndrome are merely two different diagnoses that can only be distinguished by a small number of biomarkers [66].

Many studies suggest that zinfandel might be valuable in treating metabolic disease. Resveratrol exhibited a more significant consequence on the metabolic disease, hepatic oxidative pressure, and insulin sensitivity in rats compared to metformin. Resveratrol therapy reduced blood cholesterol, C-reactive protein, and body mass indices in a pig model. These findings suggest that resveratrol has a beneficial effect on metabolic syndrome risk variables [67]. Resveratrol has the potential to improve cardiovascular health while easing the burden of chronic metabolic disease. In the mice used in the other metabolic syndrome animal model, zinfandel treatment was found to have a positive effect on the liver and skeletal muscle glucose metabolism and result in better control of glucose points [68].

5. Challenges and future perspectives

It has been investigated if resveratrol, a well-known polyphenolic stilbene, may be used to treat a variability of neoplasms, counting B-cell malignancies. It now appears to be a promising molecule for prospective therapeutic usage due to its extensive accessibility and versatility [25].

Forecasts based on epidemiological data from Western Europe and the United States suggest that a low rate of systemic treatment initiation would result in an increase in patients. Moreover, the increased prevalence may be linked to an aging population, toxicity brought on by the accumulation of treatment drugs over time, and an increase in the probability of recurrence [69]. Also, it is vital to understand the genetic influences that subsidize the expansion of disease. Non-Hodgkin lymphoma and autoimmune illnesses are both caused by inherited factors, according to a study by Din et al. An overlay of jeopardy influences may designate that cancer may develop if these genetic abnormalities are not addressed [25]. In a different study, Chang et al. [70] looked into the relationship between hematological malignancies and family history. Despite the absence of a clear link to environmental factors, a significant increase in the risk of incidence persisted if a first-degree relative had a history of cancer by genetics as well. Despite being large wine consumers, these nations have a superior prevalence of B-cell malignancies than the respite of the ecosphere. Resveratrol's low solubility and stability, which have been demonstrated to directly influence its bioavailability, may be a significant factor. To address these obstacles, new treatment strategies are being used, although development is still sluggish. To prevent the onset of disease and improve the effectiveness of therapy, it has been acknowledged that a variability of aspects in accumulation to alimentary supplements need to be looked at. The factors mentioned above could have a big impact on this [51].

Several pre-clinical studies have been carried out to evaluate the pharmacological effects of resveratrol; nevertheless, significant improvements in clinical research are still needed. This necessitates thorough evaluations of the protection and noxiousness silhouette of this substance, taking into account its connections with additional phytochemicals and synthetic anticancer drugs, as well as clinical study in a range of groups [71]. Its natural sources provide a number of formulation difficulties, including truncated solubility and long-term constancy, for instance, fast universal metabolism, which limits its distribution to aim muscles and affects its absorption. In the end, this makes it more challenging to get the desired therapeutic benefits. Moreover, resveratrol prescription has resulted in nephrotoxicity in multiple myeloma patients; the danger of toxicity linked through abiding dosage for chronic conditions must thus be carefully considered. Before extending its investigation as a possible anticancer drug and opening up new possibilities for diverse usage, these difficulties must be solved [4].

The bioavailability of this drug has been enhanced using a number of nano-strategies as the emphasis on nano technical distribution endures to produce. To overcome problems with medication delivery optimization, several strategies are being employed. The authors have highlighted many of these therapeutic methods to stimulate conversation on the value of these nanoformulations. The poor potency of current preparations is a huge unfulfilled need that could potentially be addressed by manufacturing resveratrol analogues, some of which have been investigated, to greatly boost its anticancer capabilities [51].

The aforementioned is important to begin the protection of resveratrol in gruesome patients, even if it has been proven to be well tolerated in healthy persons at both short- and long-term dosages. Further focused clinical trials with a wider variety of demographics are necessary to completely understand the safety and effectiveness of this chemical by way of its pharmacological probable [51].

6. Conclusion

Using botanical compounds to ward against or perhaps remedy illnesses has grown in popularity in recent years. Resveratrol is a cheap, accessible, and simple-to-acquire small molecule that can be functionalized. It has a variety of pharmacological actions and is not poisonous, making it suitable for industrial application. This chapter focuses on the research of new resveratrol developments, emphasizing the substance's botanical supplies, production techniques, customization, and possible therapeutic applications. Several protective benefits of resveratrol are seen in CVDs. They include actions that reduce the risk of atherosclerosis, reduce inflammation, lower blood pressure, promote cardio protection, and alter metabolism. With more investigation, it could be viable to employ resveratrol in the diagnosis or prophylaxis of CVDs. For example, we propose that resveratrol might be administered as a preventive medication to individuals with coronary artery hypertension undergoing stent placement, aiming to mitigate complications and reduce mortality associated with the procedure. Resveratrol impersonates calorie constraint in yeast by activating Sirt2, increasing DNA integrity, and lengthening life distance, which substantially implies that this substance might have additional significant impacts on adult wellness.

Acknowledgements

Authors are thankful to the Government College University for providing literature collection facilities. We confirm the final authorship for this manuscript, and we ensure that anyone else who contributed to the manuscript but does not qualify for authorship has been acknowledged with their permission. We acknowledge that all listed authors have made a significant scientific contribution to the research in the manuscript, approved its claims, and agreed to be an author.

Funding

The authors declare that no funds, grants, or other support were received during the preparation of this manuscript.

Conflict of interest

Authors declare that they have no conflict of interest.

Ethical approval

This article does not contain any studies with human participants or animals performed by any of the authors.

Consent to participate

Corresponding and all the co-authors are willing to participate in this manuscript.

Consent for publication

All authors are willing for publication of this manuscript.

Data availability

Even though adequate data has been given in the form of tables and figures, however, all authors declare that if more data required then the data will be provided on request basis.

Author details

Fakhar Islam[1,2], Umber Shehzadi[1], Farhan Saeed[1], Rabia Shabir Ahmad[1], Muhammad Umair Arshad[1], Muhammad Sadiq Naseer[3], Fatima Tariq[3], Rehman Ali[1], Sadaf Khurshid[4], Ghulam Hussain[5], Aftab Ahmad[6], Muhammad Afzaal[1], Rabia Akram[5], Osman Tuncay Agar[7], Ali Imran[1,7]* and Hafiz A.R. Suleria[7]

1 Department of Food Science, Government College University, Faisalabad, Pakistan

2 Department of Food Science and Technology, NUR International University, Lahore, Pakistan

3 Department of Clinical Nutrition, NUR International University, Lahore, Pakistan

4 Department of Home Economics, Government College University, Faisalabad, Pakistan

5 Neurochemicalbiology and Genetics Laboratory (NGL), Faculty of Life Sciences, Department of Physiology, Government College University, Faisalabad, Pakistan

6 Department of Nutritional Science, Government College University, Faisalabad, Pakistan

7 School of Agriculture, Food and Ecosystem Sciences, Faculty of Science, The University of Melbourne, Parkville, VIC, Australia

*Address all correspondence to: aliimran.ft@gmail.com; imran.a@unimelb.edu.au

References

[1] Wijekoon HS, Kim S, Bwalya EC, Fang J, Aoshima K, Hosoya K, et al. Anti-arthritic effect of pentosan polysulfate in rats with collagen-induced arthritis. Research in Veterinary Science. 2019;**122**:179-185

[2] Vestergaard M, Ingmer H. Antibacterial and antifungal properties of resveratrol. International Journal of Antimicrobial Agents. 2019;**53**(6):716-723

[3] Elshaer M, Chen Y, Wang XJ, Tang X. Resveratrol: An overview of its anti-cancer mechanisms. Life Sciences. 2018;**207**:340-349

[4] Wu S-X, Xiong R-G, Huang S-Y, Zhou D-D, Saimaiti A, Zhao C-N, et al. Effects and mechanisms of resveratrol for prevention and management of cancers: An updated review. Critical Reviews in Food Science and Nutrition. 2022;**63**:12422-12440

[5] Patra S, Mishra SR, Behera BP, Mahapatra KK, Panigrahi DP, Bhol CS, et al. Autophagy-modulating phytochemicals in cancer therapeutics: Current evidences and future perspectives. Seminars in Cancer Biology. 2022;**80**:205-217

[6] Kashyap D, Tuli HS, Yerer MB, Sharma A, Sak K, Srivastava S, et al. Natural product-based nanoformulations for cancer therapy: Opportunities and challenges. Seminars in Cancer Biology. 2021;**69**:5-23

[7] Abadi AJ, Mirzaei S, Mahabady MK, Hashemi F, Zabolian A, Hashemi F, et al. Curcumin and its derivatives in cancer therapy: Potentiating antitumor activity of cisplatin and reducing side effects. Phytotherapy Research. 2022;**36**(1):189-213

[8] Denlinger N, Bond D, Jaglowski S. CAR T-cell therapy for B-cell lymphoma. Current Problems in Cancer. 2022;**46**(1):100826

[9] Wang G-Z, Shang R, Cheng W-M, Fu Y. Irradiation-induced heck reaction of unactivated alkyl halides at room temperature. Journal of the American Chemical Society. 2017;**139**(50):18307-18312

[10] Wang G-Z, Shang R, Fu Y. Irradiation-induced palladium-catalyzed decarboxylative heck reaction of aliphatic N-(acyloxy) phthalimides at room temperature. Organic Letters. 2018;**20**(3):888-891

[11] Martínez AV, García JI, Mayoral JA. An expedient synthesis of resveratrol through a highly recoverable palladium catalyst. Tetrahedron. 2017;**73**(38):5581-5584

[12] Andrus MB, Liu J. Synthesis of polyhydroxylated ester analogs of the stilbene resveratrol using decarbonylative heck couplings. Tetrahedron Letters. 2006;**47**(32):5811-5814

[13] Perin G, Barcellos AM, Luz EQ, Borges EL, Jacob RG, Lenardão EJ, et al. Green hydroselenation of aryl alkynes: Divinyl selenides as a precursor of resveratrol. Molecules. 2017;**22**(2):327

[14] Uzura S, Sekine-Suzuki E, Nakanishi I, Sonoda M, Tanimori S. A facile and rapid access to resveratrol derivatives and their radioprotective activity. Bioorganic & Medicinal Chemistry Letters. 2016;**26**(16):3886-3891

[15] Solladié G, Pasturel-Jacopé Y, Maignan J. A re-investigation of resveratrol synthesis by Perkins

reaction. Application to the synthesis of aryl cinnamic acids. Tetrahedron. 2003;**59**(18):3315-3321

[16] Alonso F, Riente P, Yus M. Synthesis of resveratrol, DMU-212 and analogues through a novel Wittig-type olefination promoted by nickel nanoparticles. Tetrahedron Letters. 2009;**50**(25):3070-3073

[17] Tian B, Liu J. Resveratrol: A review of plant sources, synthesis, stability, modification and food application. Agriculture. 2020;**100**(4):1392-1404

[18] Aissa C. Mechanistic manifold and new developments of the Julia–Kocienski reaction. European Journal of Organic Chemistry. 2009;**2009**(12):1831-1844

[19] Gómez Baraibar Á, Reichert D, Mügge C, Seger S, Gröger H, Kourist R. A one-pot cascade reaction combining an encapsulated decarboxylase with a metathesis catalyst for the synthesis of bio-based antioxidants. Angewandte Chemie (International Ed. in English). 2016;**55**(47):14823-14827

[20] Goh YL, Cui YT, Pendharkar V, Adsool VA. Toward resolving the resveratrol conundrum: Synthesis and *in vivo* pharmacokinetic evaluation of BCP–resveratrol. ACS Medicinal Chemistry Letters. 2017;**8**(5):516-520

[21] Chung JH, Lee J-S, Lee HGJC, Biointerfaces SB. Resveratrol-loaded chitosan–γ-poly (glutamic acid) nanoparticles: Optimization, solubility, UV stability, and cellular antioxidant activity. Colloids and Surfaces. B, Biointerfaces. 2020;**186**:110702

[22] Dhakar NK, Matencio A, Caldera F, Argenziano M, Cavalli R, Dianzani C, et al. Comparative evaluation of solubility, cytotoxicity and photostability studies of resveratrol and oxyresveratrol loaded nanosponges. Pharmaceutics. 2019;**11**(10):545

[23] Sarma S, Agarwal S, Bhuyan P, Hazarika J, Ganguly M. Resveratrol-loaded chitosan–pectin core–shell nanoparticles as novel drug delivery vehicle for sustained release and improved antioxidant activities. Royal Society Open Science. 2022;**9**(2):210784

[24] Spogli R, Bastianini M, Ragonese F, Iannitti RG, Monarca L, Bastioli F, et al. Solid dispersion of resveratrol supported on magnesium dihydroxide (resv@mdh) microparticles improves oral bioavailability. Nutrients. 2018;**10**(12):1925

[25] Ioniță S, Lincu D, Mitran R-A, Ziko L, Sedky NK, Deaconu M, et al. Resveratrol encapsulation and release from pristine and functionalized mesoporous silica carriers. Pharmaceutics. 2022;**14**(1):203

[26] Yi J, He Q, Peng G, Fan Y. Improved water solubility, chemical stability, antioxidant and anticancer activity of resveratrol via nanoencapsulation with pea protein nanofibrils. Food Chemistry. 2022;**377**:131942

[27] Zhai L, Zhang Z, Guo L, Dong H, Yu J, Zhang G. Gefitinib-resveratrol cocrystal with optimized performance in dissolution and stability. Journal of Pharmaceutical Sciences. 2022;**111**(12):3224-3231

[28] Jeong SH, Hanh TM, Kim HK, Lee SR, Song I-S, Noh SJ, et al. HS-1793, a recently developed resveratrol analogue protects rat heart against hypoxia/reoxygenation injury via attenuating mitochondrial damage. Bioorganic & Medicinal Chemistry Letters. 2013;**23**(14):4225-4229

[29] Laza-Knoerr AL, Gref R, Couvreur P. Cyclodextrins for drug delivery. Journal of Drug Targeting. 2010;**18**(9):645-656

[30] Delmas D, Aires V, Limagne E, et al. Transport, stability, and biological activity of resveratrol. Annals of the New York Academy of Sciences. 2011;**1215**:48-59

[31] Jannin B, Menzel M, Berlot J-P, Delmas D, Lançon A, Latruffe N. Transport of resveratrol, a cancer chemopreventive agent, to cellular targets: Plasmatic protein binding and cell uptake. Biochemical Pharmacology. 2004;**68**:1113-1118

[32] Wang P, Sang S. Metabolism and pharmacokinetics of resveratrol and pterostilbene. BioFactors. 2018;**44**(1):16-25

[33] Miksits M, Maier-Salamon A, Aust S, Thalhammer T, Reznicek G, Kunert O, et al. Sulfation of resveratrol in human liver: Evidence of a major role for the sulfotransferases SULT1A1 and SULT1E1. Xenobiotica. 2005;**35**(12):1101-1119

[34] Jhou J-P, Chen S-J, Huang H-Y, Lin W-W, Huang D-Y, Tzeng S-J. Upregulation of FcγRIIB by resveratrol via NF-κB activation reduces B-cell numbers and ameliorates lupus. Experimental & Molecular Medicine. 2017;**49**(9):e381-e381

[35] Lee-Chang C, Bodogai M, Martin-Montalvo A, Wejksza K, Sanghvi M, Moaddel R, et al. Inhibition of breast cancer metastasis by resveratrol-mediated inactivation of tumor-evoked regulatory B cells. Journal of Immunology. 2013;**191**(8):4141-4151

[36] Galiniak S, Aebisher D, Bartusik-Aebisher D. Health benefits of resveratrol administration. Acta Biochimica Polonica. 2019;**66**(1):13-21

[37] Wu Z, Liu B, Liu J, Zhang Q, Liu J, Chen N, et al. Resveratrol inhibits the proliferation of human melanoma cells by inducing G1/S cell cycle arrest and apoptosis. Molecular Medicine Reports. 2015;**11**(1):400-404

[38] Ruan B-F, Lu X-Q, Song J, Zhu H-L. Derivatives of resveratrol: Potential agents in prevention and treatment of cardiovascular disease. Current Medicinal Chemistry. 2012;**19**(24):4175-4183

[39] He S, Yan X. From resveratrol to its derivatives: New sources of natural antioxidant. Current Medicinal Chemistry. 2013;**20**(8):1005-1017

[40] Li T, Guo Q, Qu Y, Li Y, Liu H, Liu L, et al. Solubility and physicochemical properties of resveratrol in peanut oil. Food Chemistry. 2022;**368**:130687

[41] Kumar A, Kurmi BD, Singh A, Singh D. Potential role of resveratrol and its nano-formulation as anti-cancer agent. Exploration of Targeted Anti-tumor Therapy. 2022;**3**(5):643

[42] Li Y, Zhang R, Zhang Q, Luo M, Lu F, He Z, et al. Dual strategy for improving the oral bioavailability of resveratrol: Enhancing water solubility and inhibiting glucuronidation. Journal of Agricultural and Food Chemistry. 2021;**69**(32):9249-9258

[43] Aviram M, Rosenblat M. Paraoxonases 1, 2, and 3, oxidative stress, and macrophage foam cell formation during atherosclerosis development. Free Radical Biology & Medicine. 2004;**37**(9):1304-1316

[44] Voloshyna I, Hai O, Littlefield MJ, Carsons S, Reiss AB. Resveratrol mediates anti-atherogenic effects on cholesterol flux in human macrophages and endothelium via PPARγ and adenosine. European Journal of Pharmacology. 2013;**698**(1-3):299-309

[45] Lin M-T, Yen M-L, Lin C-Y, Kuo M-L. Inhibition of vascular endothelial growth factor-induced angiogenesis by resveratrol through interruption of Src-dependent

vascular endothelial cadherin tyrosine phosphorylation. Molecular Pharmacology. 2003;**64**(5):1029-1036

[46] Donato AJ, Eskurza I, Silver AE, Levy AS, Pierce GL, Gates PE, et al. Direct evidence of endothelial oxidative stress with aging in humans: Relation to impaired endothelium-dependent dilation and upregulation of nuclear factor-κB. Circulation Research. 2007;**100**(11):1659-1666

[47] Gurusamy N, Ray D, Lekli I, Das DK. Red wine antioxidant resveratrol-modified cardiac stem cells regenerate infarcted myocardium. Journal of Cellular and Molecular Medicine. 2010;**14**(9):2235-2239

[48] Zhang H, Morgan B, Potter BJ, Ma L, Dellsperger KC, Ungvari Z, et al. Resveratrol improves left ventricular diastolic relaxation in type 2 diabetes by inhibiting oxidative/nitrative stress: *In vivo* demonstration with magnetic resonance imaging. American Journal of Physiology. Heart and Circulatory Physiology. 2010;**299**(4):H985-H994

[49] Hsu C-N, Hou C-Y, Chang-Chien G-P, Lin S, Chan JY, Lee C-T, et al. Maternal resveratrol therapy protected adult rat offspring against hypertension programmed by combined exposures to asymmetric dimethylarginine and trimethylamine-N-oxide. The Journal of Nutritional Biochemistry. 2021;**93**:108630

[50] Huang X, Liu Y, Zou Y, Liang X, Peng Y, McClements DJ, et al. Encapsulation of resveratrol in zein/pectin core-shell nanoparticles: Stability, bioaccessibility, and antioxidant capacity after simulated gastrointestinal digestion. Food Hydrocolloids. 2019;**93**:261-269

[51] Gupta DS, Gadi V, Kaur G, Chintamaneni M, Tuli HS, Ramniwas S, et al. Resveratrol and its role in the management of B-cell malignancies—A recent update. Biomedicine. 2023;**11**(1):221

[52] Pauluk D, Padilha AK, Khalil NM, Mainardes RM. Chitosan-coated zein nanoparticles for oral delivery of resveratrol: Formation, characterization, stability, mucoadhesive properties and antioxidant activity. Food Hydrocolloids. 2019;**94**:411-417

[53] Zhang F, Khan MA, Cheng H, Liang L. Co-encapsulation of α-tocopherol and resveratrol within zein nanoparticles: Impact on antioxidant activity and stability. Journal of Food Engineering. 2019;**247**:9-18

[54] Zhao W, Li A, Feng X, Hou T, Liu K, Liu B, et al. Metformin and resveratrol ameliorate muscle insulin resistance through preventing lipolysis and inflammation in hypoxic adipose tissue. Cell Signaling. 2016;**28**(9):1401-1411

[55] Fogacci F, Tocci G, Presta V, Fratter A, Borghi C, Cicero AFG. Effect of resveratrol on blood pressure: A systematic review and meta-analysis of randomized, controlled, clinical trials. Critical Reviews in Food Science and Nutrition. 2019;**59**(10):1605-1618

[56] Liu Y, Ma W, Zhang P, He S, Huang D. Effect of resveratrol on blood pressure: A meta-analysis of randomized controlled trials. Clinical Nutrition. 2015;**34**(1):27-34

[57] Marques BCAA, Trindade M, Aquino JCF, Cunha AR, Gismondi RO, Neves MF, et al. Beneficial effects of acute trans-resveratrol supplementation in treated hypertensive patients with endothelial dysfunction. Clinical and Experimental Hypertension. 2018;**40**(3):218-223

[58] Hoseini A, Namazi G, Farrokhian A, Reiner Ž, Aghadavod E, Bahmani F, et al.

The effects of resveratrol on metabolic status in patients with type 2 diabetes mellitus and coronary heart disease. Food and Function. 1 Sep 2019;**10**(9):6042-6051. DOI: 10.1039/c9fo01075k. Epub 2019 September 5. PMID: 31486447

[59] Liu F, Ma D, Luo X, Zhang Z, He L, Gao Y, et al. Fabrication and characterization of protein-phenolic conjugate nanoparticles for co-delivery of curcumin and resveratrol. Food Hydrocolloids. 2018a;**79**:450-461

[60] Torres V, Hamdi M, Millán de la Blanca M, Urrego R, Echeverri J, López-Herrera A, et al. Resveratrol–cyclodextrin complex affects the expression of genes associated with lipid metabolism in bovine *in vitro* produced embryos. Reproduction in Domestic Animals. 2018;**53**(4):850-858

[61] Liu R, Dai L, Zou Z, Si C. Drug-loaded poly (L-lactide)/lignin stereocomplex film for enhancing stability and sustained release of trans-resveratrol. International Journal of Biological Macromolecules. 2018b;**119**:1129-1136

[62] da Silva R, Teixeira JA, Nunes WDG, Zangaro GAC, Pivatto M, Caires FJ, et al. Resveratrol: A thermoanalytical study. Food Chemistry. 2017;**237**:561-565

[63] Liang Q, Ren X, Zhang X, Hou T, Chalamaiah M, Ma H, et al. Effect of ultrasound on the preparation of resveratrol-loaded zein particles. Journal of Food Engineering. 2018;**221**:88-94

[64] Pineda-Sanabria SE, Robertson IM, Sykes BD. Structure of trans-resveratrol in complex with the cardiac regulatory protein troponin C. Biochemistry. 2011;**50**(8):1309-1320

[65] Chan GG, Koch CM, Connors LH. Blood proteomic profiling in inherited (ATTRm) and acquired (ATTRwt) forms of transthyretin-associated cardiac amyloidosis. Journal of Proteome Research. 2017;**16**(4):1659-1668

[66] Singh D, Mendonsa R, Koli M, Subramanian M, Nayak SK. Antibacterial activity of resveratrol structural analogues: A mechanistic evaluation of the structure-activity relationship. Toxicology and Applied Pharmacology. 2019;**367**:23-32

[67] Chalal M, Vervandier-Fasseur D, Meunier P, Cattey H, Hierso J-C. Syntheses of polyfunctionalized resveratrol derivatives using Wittig and heck protocols. Tetrahedron. 2012;**68**(20):3899-3907

[68] Fang J-G, Zhou B. Structure–activity relationship and mechanism of the tocopherol-regenerating activity of resveratrol and its analogues. Journal of Agricultural and Food Chemistry. 2008;**56**(23):11458-11463

[69] Kanas G, Ge W, Quek RG, Keeven K, Nersesyan K, Arnason JE. Epidemiology of diffuse large B-cell lymphoma (DLBCL) and follicular lymphoma (FL) in the United States and Western Europe: Population-level projections for 2020-2025. Leukemia & Lymphoma. 2022;**63**(1):54-63

[70] Chang ET, Smedby KE, Hjalgrim H, Porwit-MacDonald A, Roos G, Glimelius B, et al. Family history of hematopoietic malignancy and risk of lymphoma. Journal of the National Cancer Institute. 2005;**97**(19):1466-1474

[71] Ashique S, Afzal O, Yasmin S, Hussain A, Altamimi MA, Webster TJ, et al. Strategic nanocarriers to control neurodegenerative disorders: Concept, challenges, and future perspective. International Journal of Pharmaceutics. 2023;**633**:122614

Section 3

Non-Food Application

Chapter 3

Resveratrol: A Promising Antiaging Agent for Cosmetic Skin Treatments

Javier Fidalgo, Ana Novo Barros and Ana Casas

Abstract

Nowadays, resveratrol, a polyphenolic phytoalexin is increasingly included in the formulas of cosmetic products and dermatology as an active ingredient, as a consequence of the well-known health beneficial properties, namely antioxidant, anti-inflammatory, anti-viral and anti-bacterial effects. This important compound can be biosynthesized naturally by plants or by industrial synthetic processes. Apart from its anti-inflammatory and antioxidant effects, a broad spectrum of effects has been attributed to the use of this compound such as anti-aging, skin-whitening, anti-angiogenic, collagen I and III stimulation (in fibroblasts) and estrogen-like effects, as well as the ability to protect cells against hydrogen peroxide-induced oxidative stress and UV-irradiation-mediated cell death. In cosmetology and dermatology has been popular because of its ability to penetrate the skin barrier and its anti-aging activity. In fact, resveratrol as an important impact on the regulation of inflammation and, as consequence, repair-related processes in skin. Furthermore, when administered either topically or orally has been proven to be safe and also to overcome the skin barrier. This review will focus in its potential application on melasma treatment and in photo-aging. Resveratrol chemistry, pharmacology, mechanism of action and evidence of its efficacy as photo skin aging protector and its potential use in melasma is discussed.

Keywords: resveratrol, cosmetic, antiaging, skin treatments, biological properties

1. Introduction

1.1 Chemistry and biological properties

Resveratrol (3,4′,5-trihydroxy-*trans*-stilbene) is a naturally occurring compound, belongs to the stilbenoid group of polyphenols, which is synthesized by plants (e.g., red grapes and berries). It can also be obtained by chemical synthesis, biotechnological synthesis or by plant extraction [1]. As observed in **Figure 1**, resveratrol consists in two phenol rings linked by an ethylene bridge, giving rise to two geometric isomers, is the biologically active *trans*-isomer and an inactive *cis*-isomer [2]. The *trans*-resveratrol can undergo photoisomerization (exposed to sun light or to artificial or natural UV radiation) to be converted into its biologically inactive *cis*-isomer [3–5].

IntechOpen

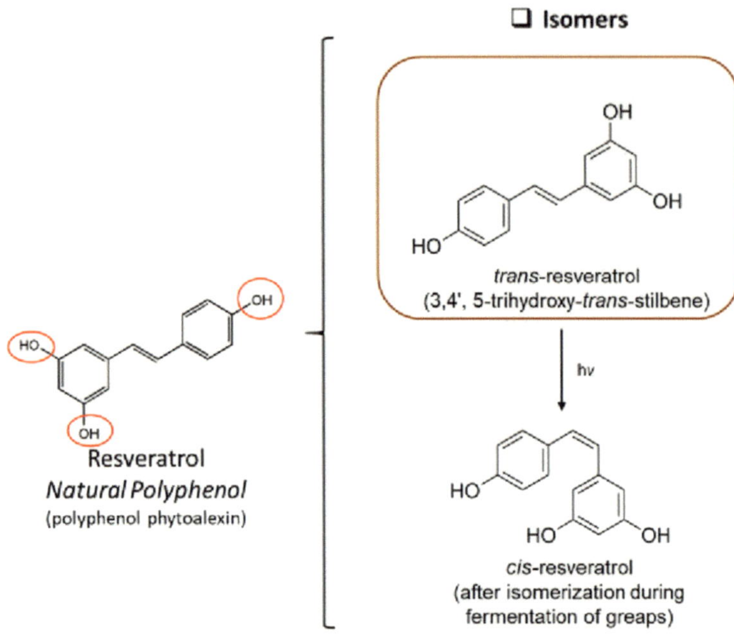

Figure 1.
Chemical structures of resveratrol and its two isomers, trans- and cis-resveratrol. Highlighted in red circles the hydroxyl groups of the phenolic moieties of resveratrol. Highlighted in a brown squared the biologically active trans-isomer.

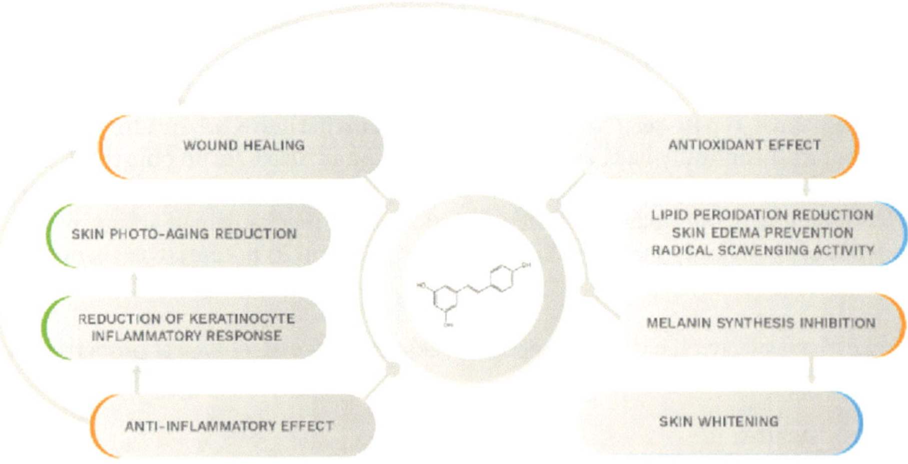

Figure 2.
Biological properties from resveratrol.

Resveratrol is a compound that presents several important biological properties, (**Figure 2**).

The aim of this study is to show the efficacy and tolerability of resveratrol, that can have a topical application to the face and to determine whether this topical treatment with resveratrol can reduce anti-aging effects by improving skin barrier, and elasticity. In fact, Andrzej et al., 2022 [6] concluded that "resveratrol shows an excellent biocompatibility" representing an interesting and promissing novel therapeutical compound for the cosmetic industry.

2. Pharmacology, toxicity and skin permeation

Orally, and considering its structure, resveratrol is rapidly absorbed from the gastrointestinal tract, but with a low bioavailability because is rapidly metabolized in the liver [2]. In human, its plasma half-life has been reported to be 9.2 ± 0.6 hours [7], resulting not carcinogenic in mouse, without developmental and reproductive toxicity [8]. Another important characteristic from this compound, is that, as already proved, it is non-irritating to skin and eyes and non-sensitizing. *In vitro* and *in vivo* resveratrol demonstrated to be nontoxic, safe for oral and dermal application, as well as being well tolerated [9–11]. Resveratrol also showed high permeability in the skin, overcoming the skin barrier in its neutral (non-ionized) form, showing that it is readily available in the stratum corneum (SC) in animal and human studies [12, 13]. This is of high importance, once the most exposure to reactive oxygen species (ROS) takes place in the SC, supporting the use of resveratrol in cosmeceuticals [14, 15].

2.1 Possible skin application in melasma and it use in skin photoaging

2.1.1 Antioxidant activity

Skin care formulations are usually based on exogenous antioxidants that cannot be synthesized by our body, like vitamins or phenolic compounds. Some studies referred in Literature, report that resveratrol is able to inhibit UV-induced lipid peroxidation. UV irradiation (UV A and B) and blue light are known to induce the formation of free radicals, reactive oxygen species (ROS; e.g., peroxides, superoxide, hydroxyl radical) *in vivo* [16–18], and these reactive oxygen species may be toxic and mutagenic. They can also negatively influence some immunological processes and aging, as well as pathophysiological mechanisms leading to skin inflammatory disorders [19]. *Melasma* was associated with the increased ROS levels which will lead to the oxidation of proteins and lipids, and causing oxidative damage to the cells [20–23]. *Skin photoaging* is also associated with ROS due to the exposure of the skin to sun light [24]. Recent studies also suggested melasma as a photoaging skin disorder [25]. Resveratrol is active in neutralizing, and inhibiting, the formation of ROS, but it also is effective in neutralizing synthetic DPPH and AAPH radicals *in vitro* [26]. Resveratrol was also proven to have radical scavenging properties owing most of it by the *para*/hydroxyl group of its structure [25, 27]. In a different study was observed to be a better antioxidant than many flavonoids [28]. For example, the antiradical activity of resveratrol relative to peroxide radicals was higher than catechins, gallic acid, and elagic acid (resveratrol> catechin> epicatechin = gallocatechin> gallic acid = ellagic acid.

In an *in vitro* study in human keratinocyte cells (HaCaT cells) after UV A radiation, considered by some authors as the major actor for the photoaging process [29], resveratrol is able to decrease oxidative by-products (e.g., maleic dialdehyde) and to increase antioxidants such as superoxide dismutase (SOD) and glutathione peroxidase (GPX) [30]. Manganese superoxide dismutase (MnSOD), a very important antioxidant enzyme, was also increased in the presence of resveratrol [31]. Compared to Vitamins A and C, it was proved to be even more effective against lipid peroxidation

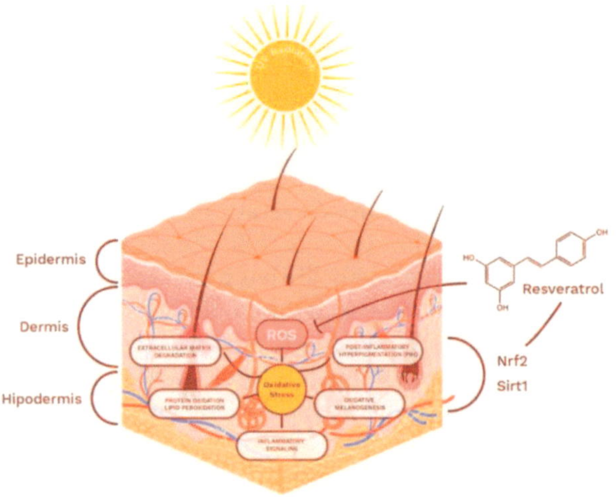

Figure 3.
Association of Resveratrol in the different biological processes triggered by UV radiation in the skin.

and protein oxidation *in vitro* [32–34], but also in an *in vivo* study in hairless mice [35]. Furthermore, DNA damage caused by peroxidyl radicals in human lymphocytes was reduced by resveratrol treatment after UV B induced H_2O_2 production [36]. Another key molecule in oxidation is the transcription factor nuclear factor-E2-related factor-2 (Nrf2) which regulates genes that help synthesize more antioxidants and remove ROS. Resveratrol upregulates Nrf2 which increase the levels of antioxidants such as GPX, SOD, catalase, and hemoxygenase [31, 37, 38]. In addition, Resveratrol activates a NAD^+-dependent protein deacetylase, SIRT-1, a protein which is involved in cell survival against oxidative stress by decreasing the ROS levels [39]. In different in vivo studies was also observed an increase in SIRT-1 following resveratrol treatment of 0.02% in the diet for 4 weeks in wild-type mice (**Figure 3**) [40].

2.1.2 Skin-whitening activity and photoaging protection

One the common clinical characteristic of melasma is the appearance of skin hyperpigmentation mainly in the face [22, 23]. In photoaging hyperpigmentation also occurs by cumulative sun exposure [41]. Resveratrol has the ability to modulate the tyrosinase activity by the inhibition of this enzyme and by acting as a competitive substrate, and thus blocking melanogenesis [42–44]. This compound also inhibits hyperpigmentation by other different mechanisms of action. According to Newton R. A. et al., 2007 [45], at a transcriptional level, resveratrol inhibits the mRNA expression of tyrosinase, tyrosinase-related proteins (Tyrp1 and Tyrp2), microphthalmia-associated transcription factor (MITF), a major regulator of melanogenesis, and DOPAchrome tautomerase (DCT) in human melanocytes *in vitro* study. On the other hand, it decreases the levels of melanin and in *in vivo* studies were observed by topically administration of resveratrol in guinea pig [46]. Resveratrol was also found effective in the inhibition of melanogenesis, (**Figure 3**).

2.1.3 Anti-inflammatory activity and collagen synthesis stimulation

Both, in melasma and skin aging, a decrease in the quantity of collagen I, III, IV-VII (decrease in collagen I, IV in melasma, and all of them in skin aging) in the dermis and basal membrane has been described. In keratinocytes UV A radiation, ROS can upregulate the AP-1 (activator protein 1) and NF-kB (nuclear factor kappa beta) transcription factors [47, 48]. Their upregulation results in the induction of matrix metalloproteinase activity leading to the interference with intracellular signaling pathways responsible to the expression of genes regulating the process of collagen type I and III, resulting in hypertrophy and degradation of elastin and hyaluronic acid [45, 48, 49]. Resveratrol was found to reduce the expression of AP-1 and NF-kB transcription factors, limiting the degradation process of collagen and elastin in the skin, but also skin inflammation [48, 50–52]. In addition, resveratrol has been to act as an NF-kB inhibitor [53] which can be activated by ROS playing and important role in the inflammatory response [54, 55].

3. Wound healing potential of resveratrol

Another interesting potential property of this substance is their application to the wound healing process. Wound healing is a natural biological mechanism of repairing tissues after suffering from an injury. After tissue damage Nrf-2 and NF-kB play a crucial role in both inflammation and oxidation processes during wound healing process [56]. On the other hand, it is suggested that ROS in not excessive, low, levels are necessary for the wound healing process to fight against pathogens invading the organism, but not good when are produced in high levels in the tissue [57]. So, a control of the ROS produced by compounds such as Resveratrol knowing its proven anti-oxidant capacity is of interest to reduce the excess of tissue damage [58]. In addition, in a work from 2006 [59] was observed the association of an increase in the expression of the VEFG (Vascular Endotelian Growth Factor) *in vitro* and *in vivo* (mice) with the increase in agiogenesis which favored an improvement of the wound healing process. Evidence which demonstrates the potential of resveratrol on treating wound healing has been published [60, 61]. In this works was demonstrated the antioxidant, anti-inflammatory properties as well as the upregulation of Sirt-1 and VEFG expressions to play an important role in the ability of the resveratrol to improve wound healing in tissues such as the skin.

To sum up, if we take into account the related inhibition of the pro-inflammatory mediators' expression, the ROS reduction ability, the scavenging properties, the increasing in angiogenesis via increasing VEFG and Sirtuins (Sirt-1), resveratrol seems to be a valuable candidate in order to both regulate and improve the wound healing process after skin damage.

4. Clinical evidence of resveratrol uses in cosmetics

The use of resveratrol in cosmetic formulas has increased in the last 15 years because of its potential biological activities described above. The use of this substance in cosmetic formulas such as a cream containing this active ingredient was studied in the work from Igielska-Kalwat [62]. In this study 20 volunteers were administrated topically on the face a cream composed by 0.007% resveratrol and with placebo (no resveratrol cream). Results after 6 weeks showed that treated patients increased skin hydration and firmness, concluding that resveratrol has moisturizing and tightening effects in skin but also safety without any sign of skin irritation. In a different work from Ferzli G. [63], a resveratrol enriched formulation which combined resveratrol with green tea polyphenols and caffeine, reduced facial redness in 13 of the 16 subjects from this study after 12 weeks study period. The other 3 subjects left were seen only to improve skin quality at the end of this study. In 2014, Farris P. [52] demonstrated also the efficacy of another resveratrol enhanced formulation (1% resveratrol, 0 1% Vitamin E and 0.5% baicalin) in the treatment of photodamaged skin. After a 12 weeks period an improvement in fine lines and wrinkles derived from photo aging processes were observed. In a similar work from 2013 [64] the efficacy on protecting the skin after UV aggression on 15 healthy volunteers was performed. In this study after repetitive UV radiation 1% resveratrol treatment after UV damage showed better protective effect even than other antioxidants alone, and logically better than placebo treated subjects.

In a different study form Moyano J.R. [65] a W/O (water in oil) cream was prepared to optimize the permeability and stability of the trans isomer of the resveratrol and study the elasticity, hydration and luminosity capacity of the formulas in 8 women ranging from 45 to 70 years old during a 30 days trial. Results suggested the efficacy of the resveratrol emulsion produced in all patients tested. The increase in all parameters studied was 20.53%, 49.70% and 6.17% for hydration, elasticity and colorimetry respectively.

5. Conclusions

As conclusion, resveratrol could be potentially effective in the treatment of several skin disorders, including diseases or signs of aging, for example. Several studies have shown important biological activity of resveratrol, especially in reconstituted skin models, skin cell cultures, or in animal models. The high activity, and efficacy, of resveratrol as both an antioxidant and a melanin synthesis inhibitor make this compound as a promising candidate for the treatment and prevention of skin aging. Despite this beneficial influence on the skin aging effects and dermal diseases, resveratrol is also effective in healing of wounds and burns. Exist similarities between melasma and skin aging (and photoaging) in terms of the hyperpigmentation, the basement membrane disruption of the skin, as well as the association with ROS owing to the UV exposure. These similarities would make resveratrol as a promising contributor for their treatment and prevention of melasma. Because the vast majority of the literature refers to the activity of resveratrol to *in vitro* studies and *in vivo* in animal models, it would be desirable more clinical evidences of its efficacy in human skin treatment.

In our opinion, resveratrol may be able to induce collagen synthesis *in vivo*, although the molecular mechanism is not clearly established. We pretend to proceed our study of this molecule, to give an added value to the potential opportunities of this compound.

Acknowledgements

The authors thanks to Dr. José Rocha from Mesosystem for the development of the pictures.

Author details

Javier Fidalgo[1,2], Ana Novo Barros[1,2*] and Ana Casas[1,2]

1 Mesosystem S.A, Rua de Júlio Dinis, Porto, Portugal

2 Mesosystem Investigação e Investimentos by Spinpark, Barco, Guimarães, Portugal

*Address all correspondence to: pca@mesosystem.com

References

[1] Fan E, Zhang K, Zhu M, Wang Q. Obtaining resveratrol: From chemical synthesis to biotechnological production. Mini-Reviews in Organic Chemistry. 2010;**7**(4):272-281

[2] Ratz-Łyko A, Arct J. Resveratrol as an active ingredient for cosmetic and dermatological applications: A review. Journal of Cosmetic and Laser Therapy. 2018:1-7. DOI: 10.1080/14764172.2018.1469767

[3] Bernard E, Britz-McKibbin P, Gernigon N. Resveratrol photoisomerization: An integrative guided-inquiry experiment. Journal of Chemical Education. 2007;**84**(7):1159-1161

[4] Chen X, He H, Wang G, Yang B, Ren W, Ma L, et al. Stereospecific determination of cisand trans-resveratrol in rat plasma by HPLC: Application to pharmacokineticstudies. Biomedical Chromatography. 2007;**21**:257-265

[5] Camont L, Cottart C-H, Rhayem Y, Nivet-Antoine V, Djelidi R, Collin F, et al. Simple spectrophotometric assessment of the trans−/cis-resveratrol ratio in aqueous solutions. Analytica Chimica Acta. 2009;**634**:121-128

[6] Hecker A. The impact of resveratrol on skin wound healing, scarring, and aging. International Wound Journal. 2022;**19**(1):9-28

[7] Walle T, Hsieh R, DeLegge MH, Oatis JE, Walle UK. High absorption but very low bioavailability of oral resveratrol in humans. Drug Metabolism and Disposition. 2004;**32**:1377-1382

[8] Brown VA, Patel KR, Viskaduraki M, Crowell JA, Perloff M, Booth TD, et al. Repeat dose study of the cancer chemopreventive agent resveratrol in healthy volunteers: Safety, pharmacokinetics, and effect on the insulin-like growth factor axis. Cancer Research. 2010;**70**:9003-9011

[9] Williams LD, Burdock GA, Edwards JA, Beck M, Bausch J. Safety studies conducted on high-purity trans-resveratrol in experimental animals. Food and Chemical Toxicology. 2009;**47**:2170-2182

[10] Cottart CH, Nivet-Antoine V, Laguillier-Morizot C, Beaudeux JL. Resveratrol bioavailability and toxicity in humans. Molecular Nutrition & Food Research. 2010;**54**(1):7-16

[11] Amri A, Chaumeil JC, Sfar S, Charrueau CJ. Administration of resveratrol: What formulation solutions to bioavailability limitations? Journal of Controlled Release. 2012;**158**:182-193

[12] Hung CF, Lin YK, Huang ZR, Fang JY. Delivery of resveratrol, a red wine polyphenol, from solutions and hydrogels via the skin. Biological & Pharmaceutical Bulletin. 2008;**31**:955-962

[13] Timmers S, Auwerx J, Schrauwen P. The journey of resveratrol from yeast to human. Aging (Albany NY). 2005;**4**:146-158

[14] Abla MJ, Banga AK. Quantification of skin penetration of antioxidants of varying lipophilicity. International Journal of Cosmetic Science. 2013;**35**(1):19-26

[15] Borek C. Molecular mechanisms in cancer induction and prevention. Environmental Health Perspectives. 1993;**101**(3):237-245

[16] Kuse Y, Ogawa K, Tsuruma K, Shimazawa M, Hara H. Damage of photoreceptor-derived cells in culture induced by light emitting diode-derived blue light. Scientific Reports. 2014;**4**:5223, 1-12

[17] Liebel F, Kaur S, Ruvolo E, Kollias N, Southall MD. Irradiation of skin with visible light induces reactive oxygen species and matrix-degrading enzymes. The Journal of Investigative Dermatology. 2012;**132**(7):1901-1907

[18] Lohan SB et al. Free radicals induced by sunlight in different spectral regions – In vivo versus ex vivo study. Experimental Dermatogology. 2016;**25**:380-385

[19] Cai H, Xie Z, Liu G, Sun X, Peng G, Lin B, et al. Isolation, identification and activities of natural antioxidants from callicarpa kwangtungensis chun. PLoS One. 2004;**9**:e93000

[20] Handel AC, Handel AC, Miot LD, Miot HA. Melasma: A clinical and epidemiological review. Anais Brasileiros de Dermatologia. 2014;**89**(5):771-782

[21] Passeron T. Melasma pathogenesis and influencing factors – An overview of the latest research. JEADV. 2013;**27**(1):5-6

[22] Lee A-Y. An updated review of melasma pathogenesis. Dermatologica sinica. 2014;**32**(4):233-239

[23] Ogbechie-Godec OA, Elbuluk N. Melasma: An up-to-date comprehensive review. Dermatology and Therapy. 2017;**7**(3):305-318

[24] Ichihashi M, Ando H, Yoshida M, Niki Y, Matsui M. Photoaging of the skin. Anti-Aging Medicine. 2009;**6**(6):46-59

[25] Passeron T, Picardo M. Melasma, a photoaging disorder. Pigment Cell & Melanoma Research. 2018;**31**(4):461-465

[26] Miura T, Muraoka S, Ikeda N, Watanabe M, Fujimoto Y. Antioxidative and prooxidative action of stilbene derivatives. Pharmacology & Toxicology. 2000;**86**:203-208

[27] Stojanović S, Sprinz H, Brede O. Efficiency and mechanism of the antioxidant action of trans-resveratrol and its analogues in the radical liposome oxidation. Archives of Biochemistry and Biophysics. 2001;**391**:79-89

[28] Yilmaz Y, Toledo RT. Major flavonoids in grape seeds and skins. Antioxidant capacity of catechin, epicatechin, and gallic acid. Journal of Agricultural and Food Chemistry. 2004;**52**:255-260

[29] Nouveau S, Agrawal D, Kohli M, Bernerd F, Misra N, Nayak CS. Skin Hyperpigmentation in Indian population: Insights and best practice. Indian Journal of Dermatology. 2016;**61**(5):487-495

[30] Chen ML, Li J, Xiao WR, et al. Protective effect of resveratrol against oxidative damage of UVA irradiated HaCaT cells. Zhong Nan Da Xue Xue Bao Yi Xue Ban. 2006;**31**(5):635-639

[31] Carrizzo A, Puca A, Damato A, Marino M, Franco E, Pompeo F, et al. Resveratrol improves vascular function in patients with hypertension and dyslipidemia by modulating NO metabolism. Hypertension. 2013;**62**:359

[32] Weber SU, Thiele JJ, Cross CE, Packer L. Vitamin C, uric acid, and glutathione gradients in murine stratum corneum and their susceptibility to ozone exposure. The Journal of Investigative Dermatology. 1999;**113**(6):1128-1132

[33] Baxter RA. Anti-aging properties of resveratrol: Review and report of a potent new antioxidant skin care formulation.

Journal of Cosmetic Dermatology. 2008;7:2

[34] Fang JG, Lu M, Chen ZH, et al. Antioxidant effects of resveratrol and its analogues against the freeradical-induced peroxidation of linoleic acid in micelles. Chemistry. 2002;**8**(18):4191-4198

[35] Afaq F, Adhami VM, Ahmad N. Prevention of short-term ultraviolet B radiation-mediated damages by resveratrol in SKH-1 hairless mice. Toxicology and Applied Pharmacology. 2003;**186**:28-37

[36] Yen GC, Duh PD, Lin CW. Effects of resveratrol and 4-hexylresorcinol on hydrogen peroxide-induced oxidative DNA damage in human lymphocytes. Free Radical Research. 2003;**37**(5):509-514

[37] Ungvari Z, Orosz Z, Rivera A, et al. Resveratrol increases vascular oxidative stress resistance. American Journal of Physiology. Heart and Circulatory Physiology. 2007;**292**(5):12

[38] Harikumar KB, Aggarwal BB. Resveratrol: A multitargeted agent for age-associated chronic diseases. Cell Cycle. 2008;**7**(8):1020-1035

[39] Kwon S-H et al. Depigmenting effect of resveratrol is dependent on FOXO3a activation without SIRT1 activation. International Journal of Molecular Sciences. 2017;**18**:1213

[40] Nakata R, Takahashi S, Inoue H. Recent advances in the study on resveratrol. Biological & Pharmaceutical Bulletin. 2012;**35**:273

[41] Flament F, Bazin R, Laquieze S, Rubert V, Simonpietri E, Piot B. Effect of the sun on visible clinical signs of aging in Caucasian skin. Clinical, Cosmetic and Investigational Dermatology. 2013;**6**:221-232

[42] Lee SY, Baek N, Nam T-g. Natural, semisynthetic and synthetic tyrosinase inhibitors. Journal of Enzyme Inhibition and Medicinal Chemistry. 2016;**31**(1):1-13

[43] Chang T-S. An updated review of tyrosinase inhibitors. International Journal of Molecular Sciences. 2009;**10**:2440-2475

[44] Loizzo MR, Tundis R, Menichini F. Natural and synthetic tyrosinase inhibitors as antibrowning agents: An update. Comprehensive Reviews in Food Science and Food Safety. 2012;**11**:378-398

[45] Newton RA, Cook AL, Roberts DW, Leonard JH, Sturm RA. Posttranscriptional regulation of melanin biosynthetic enzymes by cAMP and resveratrol in human melanocytes. The Journal of Investigative Dermatology. 2007;**127**:2216-2227

[46] Lee TH, Seo JO, Baek SH, Kim SY. Inhibitory effects of resveratrol on melanin synthesis in ultraviolet B-induced pigmentation in guinea pig skin. Biomolecules & Therapeutics (Seoul). 2014;**22**:35-40

[47] Adhami VM, Afaq F, Ahmad N. Suppression of ultraviolet B exposure-mediated activation of NF-kappaB in normal human keratinocytes by resveratrol. Neoplasia. 2003;**5**(1):74-82

[48] Kundu JK, Shin YK, Surh YJ. Resveratrol modulates phorbol ester-induced pro-inflammatory signal transduction pathways in mouse skin in vivo: NF-kappaB and AP-1 as prime targets. Biochemical Pharmacology. 2006;**72**(11):1506-1515

[49] Petrat F, de Groot H. Protection against severe intestinal ischemia/reperfusion injury in rats by intravenous resveratrol. The Journal of Surgical Research. 2011;**167**(2):29

[50] Sen CK, Khanna S, Gordillo G, Bagchi D, Bagchi M, Roy S. Oxygen, oxidants, and antioxidants in wound healing: An emerging paradigm. Annals of the New York Academy of Sciences. 2002;**957**:239-249

[51] Leighton F, Cuevas A, Guasch V, Perez DD, Strobel P, San MA, et al. Plasma polyphenols and antioxidants, oxidative DNA damage and endothelial function in a diet and wine intervention study in humans. Drugs under Experimental and Clinical Research. 1999;**25**:133

[52] Farris P, Krutmann J, Li Y-H, McDaniel D, Krolj Y. Resveratrol: A unique antioxidant offering a multi-mechanistic approach for treating aging skin. Journal of Drugs in Dermatology. 2013;**12**:1389

[53] Nam N-H. Naturally occurring NF-Kb inhibitors. Mini-Reviews in Medicinal Chemistry. 2006;**6**: 945-951

[54] Lawrence T. The nuclear factor NF-kappaB pathway in inflammation. Cold Spring Harbor Perspectives in Biology. 2009;**1**(6):a001651

[55] Wang T, Zhang X, Jian LJ. The nuclear factor NF-kappaB pathway in inflammation. International Immunopharmacology. 2002;**2**(11):1509-1520

[56] Ambrozova N, Ulrichova J, Galandakova A. Models for the study of skin wound healing. The role of Nrf2 and NF-κB. Biomedical Papers of the Medical Faculty of the University Palacky, Olomouc, Czech Republic. 2017;**161**(1):1-13

[57] Cano SM, Lancel S, Boulanger E, Neviere R. Targeting oxidative stress and mitochondrial dysfunction in the treatment of impaired wound healing: A systematic review. Antioxidants. 2018;7(8):98

[58] Bilgen F, Ural A, Kurutas EB, Bekerecioglu M. The excess of oxidative stress and Raftlin levels on woundn healing. International Wound Journal. 2019;**16**(5):1178-1184

[59] Kanno Y et al. Lack ofa2-antiplasmin improves cutaneous wound healing viaover-released vascular endothelial growth factor-inducedangiogenesis in wound lesions. Journal of Thrombosis and Haemostasis. 2006;**4**(7):1602-1610

[60] Zhou X, Ruan Q, Ye Z, Chu Z, et al. Resveratrol accelerates wound healing by attenuating oxidative stress-induced impairment of cell proliferation and migration. Burns. 2021;**47**(1):133-139

[61] Farris P, Yatskayer M, Chen N, Krol Y, Oresajo C. Evaluation of efficacy and tolerance of a nighttime topical antioxidant containing resveratrol, baicalin, and vitamin e for treatment of mild to moderately photodamaged skin. Journal of Drugs in Dermatology. 2014;**13**(12):1467-1472

[62] Igielska-Kalwat J, Firlej F, Lewandowska A, Biedziak B. In vivo studies of resveratrol contained in cosmetic emulsions. Acta Biochimica Polonica. 2019;**66**(3):371-374

[63] Ferzli G, Patel M, Phrsai N, Brody N. Reduction of facial redness with resveratrol added to topical product containing green tea polyphenols and caffeine. Journal of Drugs in Dermatology. 2013;**12**:770-774

[64] Wu Y, Jia LL, Zheng YN, Xu XG, Luo YJ, Wang B, et al. Resveratrate protects human skin from damage due to repetitive ultraviolet irradiation.

Journal of the European Academy of Dermatology and Venereology. 2013;**27**:345-350

[65] Moyano JR, Fabbrocini G, de Stefano D, Mazzella C. Enhanced antioxidant effect of trans-resveratrol: Potential of binary systems with polyethylene glycol and cyclodextrin. Drug Development and Industrial Pharmacy. 2013;**40**(10):1-8

Section 4

Theraputic Application

Chapter 4

Resveratrol, Multiple Bioactivities for a Wide Range of Health Benefits – New Innovative Extracts for Nutraceutical, Pharmaceutical, and Cosmetics Applications

Veronique Traynard

Abstract

Resveratrol (trans-resveratrol or 3,4′,5-trihydroxystilbene) is a polyphenol naturally present in grape skin and seeds. New innovative concentrated extracts produced by microorganisms or with innovative, ecological extraction techniques allow a new generation of high-quality ingredients for a diversity of product applications in nutraceuticals, cosmetics, and pharmaceuticals. Resveratrol exerts antioxidant and anti-inflammatory properties while promoting sirtuins 1 activities and mitochondrial functions. It also modulates multiple cellular signaling molecules, such as VEGF, caspases, cytokines NF-kB, vascular cell adhesion molecule, IGF-1, PPARs, and COX-2. Its clinical benefits have been demonstrated mainly in cognitive health, menopause, bone health, cardiovascular health, glucose metabolism, sport nutrition, and skin health. This chapter reviews the bioactivities of resveratrol, its clinical benefits, and detail its potential applications in several product categories in the growing field of health and nutrition product innovation. Resveratrol-based products may participate to provide new natural and complementary solutions for a global approach to health support and maintenance.

Keywords: resveratrol, SIRT1, mitochondria, cardiovascular health, metabolic health, obesity, menopause, diabetes 2

1. Introduction

Resveratrol (3,5,4′-trans-trihydroxystilbene) is a polyphenolic phytoalexin, which enters into the stilbene category. It is a naturally occurring molecule that is commonly found in grape skin and seeds but is also present in wines and various other types of plant-based conventional foods, especially tea or berries. Resveratrol possesses two phenol rings (monophenol and diphenol) bonded together by a double styrene bond, and it exists in both cis and trans isomeric

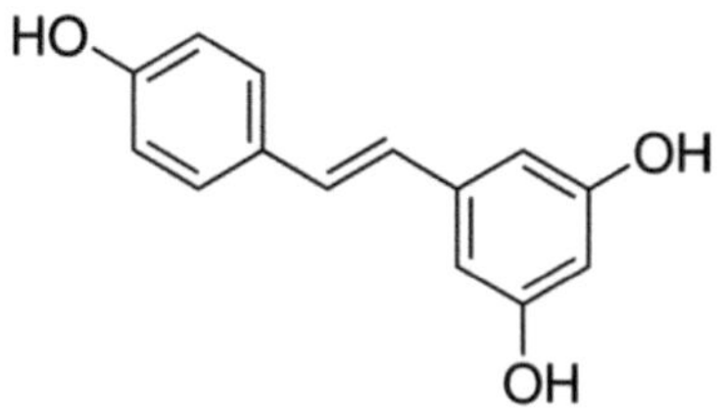

Figure 1.
Resveratrol chemical structure.

forms (**Figure 1**). Trans-resveratrol appears to be the more abundant and stable natural form for several months [1].

2. Resveratrol modulates a wide range of cellular pathways, which triggers multiple bioactivities relevant to human health

2.1 Antioxidant properties

Oxidative stress is defined as an imbalance between the generation of reactive oxygen species and the antioxidant defense system of the body in favor of oxidant production (**Figure 2**). Enhanced oxidative stress damages macromolecules, DNA, and cellular activities, and impairs cell metabolism, which underlies several age-related diseases, including cancer, diabetes, chronic kidney disease, and cardiovascular and neurodegenerative diseases. Overproduction of reactive oxygen species (ROS) induces inflammation, dysregulation of mitochondria, and cell death. Resveratrol has an inhibitory effect on excessive ROS production, aberrant mitochondrial distribution, and lipid peroxidation [2, 3]. Resveratrol decreases ROS production in epidermal keratinocytes [4] astroglial cells and prevents hepatic steatosis in HFD-induced obese mice by reducing chronic inflammation and oxidative stress [5]. Resveratrol intake by diabetic rats at a dose of 5 mg/kg/day leads to normalization of antioxidant status, exacerbated by oxidative stress induced by hyperglycemia [6]. Resveratrol also attenuates oxidative stress in rats with experimental periodontitis [7], induced early Alzheimer's disease [8], and chronic obstructive pulmonary disease [9].

2.2 Anti-inflammatory action

Resveratrol suppresses IL-6 production and secretion by macrophages [10]. Moreover, the administration of resveratrol to monocyte cultures leads to a decrease in the expression of inflammatory mediators, such as TNF-α and IL-8, without triggering cytotoxicity [11]. Resveratrol is involved in the inhibition of toll-like receptors (TLR), which in their active form may modulate proinflammatory cytokines production and chemokine expression, and stimulate the activation of innate and adaptive immunity [12]. Resveratrol reduces matrix-metalloprotease (MMP) expression and suppresses the production of IL-1, IL-6, and TNF-α in a dose-dependent manner in chondrocytes in a model of osteoarthritis. Resveratrol effectively inhibits NF-κB signaling by inhibiting the activity of NF-κB, as well as by suppressing the phosphorylation of JAK/STAT signaling pathways [13]. The supplementation with 500 mg resveratrol is associated with a reduction of the levels of proinflammatory mediators and the inhibition of NF-kB activity in patients with active ulcerative colitis, a

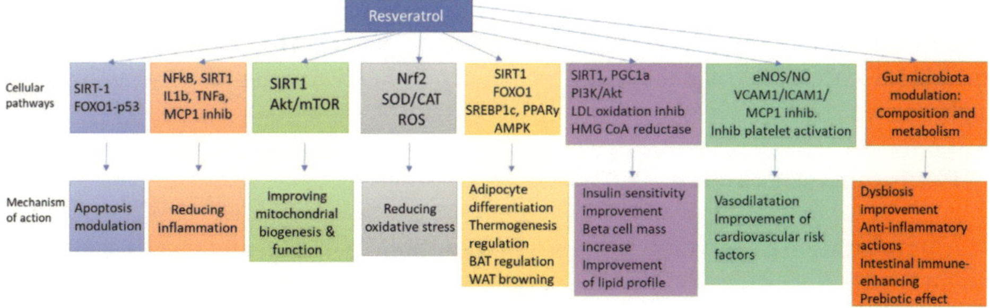

Figure 2.
Main cellular pathways modulated by resveratrol and mechanisms of actions involved.

chronic intestinal inflammatory disease [14]. The activation of the sirtuin 1 pathway by resveratrol triggers the decrease in NF-kB-induced pro-inflammatory mediators' levels, such as TNF-a, IL1b, IL6, MMP-1, MMP-3, and COX-2.

Macrophages differentiate from blood monocytes and participate in both innate and adaptative immunity. Resveratrol triggers an anti-inflammatory profile in macrophages. Several studies demonstrated that resveratrol exerts anti-inflammatory effects by attenuating TLR4-TRAF6, mitogen-activated protein kinase (MAPK), and AKT pathways in LPS-induced macrophages. Another signaling pathway that has been linked to inflammation is the endoplasmic reticulum (ER) response. More recently, it was shown that resveratrol prevents the increase of acetylated α-tubulin caused by mitochondrial damage in macrophages stimulated with inducers of the nod-like receptor family, pyrin domain containing 3 (NLRP3) [15]. It may also dose-dependently increase NK cell activity considered a primary line of defense in innate immunity [12].

Resveratrol also strongly reduces the production of granulocyte-macrophage colony-stimulating factor (GM-CSF), a pro-inflammatory cytokine that acts at the interface between innate and adaptive immunity essential for survival, the differentiation and activation of pro-inflammatory macrophages, and a key marker of atheroma formation.

2.3 Anti-glycation activity

Glycation is a chemical reaction between reducing sugars and proteins, leading to the synthesis of advanced glycation end products (AGEs) molecules. They accumulate and trigger damage at cellular levels, including endothelial dysfunction, abnormal cellular activity, alterations of protein conformation, and lipid peroxidation. Increased glycation is associated with a higher prevalence of diabetes and related complications and is also present in neurodegenerative diseases. Glycation forms highly reactive dicarbonyl compounds, such as methylglyoxal and glyoxal, which are key precursors to the production of AGE, enhancing oxidative stress in the tissues. Resveratrol supplementation in drinking water to chronic MG-treated rats significantly reduces the level of advanced oxidation protein products (AOPP), AGEs, and protein carbonyl in plasma, as well as markers of oxidative stress in the liver [16]. Moreover, resveratrol at doses ranging from 1 to 100 μM displays a protective effect in endothelial cells exposed to a high glucose-induced damage challenge. Resveratrol also inhibits the production of methylglyoxal-induced endothelial alterations by the stimulation of eNOS in the thoracic aorta in aging rodent model. Resveratrol prevents opacification and formation of polyols in the bovine lens, and improves kidney function due to suppression of AGEs formation, suggesting that resveratrol may be considered a protective agent against diabetic complications, such as cataracts and nephropathy [17, 18].

2.4 Neuroprotective action

Administration of resveratrol improves cognition, learning, and memory in a rodent model of vascular dementia. This preliminary result constitutes an interesting and encouraging finding in cognitive health and healthy aging areas [19]. Resveratrol also improves cognition and induces neuroprotection in amyloid and tau pathologies in mice models of Alzheimer's disease [20]. Resveratrol displays a neuroprotective effect in a rodent model of cerebral ischemia/reperfusion injury. Resveratrol supplementation decreases the cerebral infract volume and activates JAK2, PI3K, or Akt expression, as well as anti-apoptotic molecules. Moreover, it also inhibits the expression of pro-apoptotic caspase-3 and Bax. Interestingly, resveratrol enhanced novel object recognition performances of aged rats. In addition, resveratrol enhanced cerebral blood flow during novel object recognition task in aged rats. Several pathways related to inflammation and oxidative stress, such as eicosanoid signaling, IL6, NO and ROS synthesis, and MIF-induced innate immunity were decreased in treated groups compared to control group [21]. Several neuroprotective actions of resveratrol have been suggested in the studies of its effects in intracerebral hemorrhage [22], cerebral neurodamage [23], and central nervous system injuries, such as stroke [24]. Moreover, additional preclinical studies confirm these findings in neuroprotective and cognitive-enhancing properties. The protection of resveratrol treatment on hippocampal plasticity and memory performance in female Balb/C mice has revealed positive preliminary results. Resveratrol induced neuronal differentiation in adult hippocampal precursor cells without affecting the proliferation *in vitro* [25]. Also, resveratrol intervention improved behavioral performance, increased the production of new neurons, elevated the population of double cortin-expressing intermediate cells, and promoted hippocampal neurogenesis *in vivo*. Furthermore, after intraventricular injection of resveratrol for 7 days, the long-term memory formation and the long-time potentiation induction from hippocampus were improved in C57BL/6 J mice, while these effects were blocked in SIRT-1 mutant [26], suggesting the neuroprotective and cognitive support is mediated through SIRT-1 signaling in the aging brain. Resveratrol-treated animals showed improved learning, memory, and mood functions. Resveratrol also increased net neurogenesis and microvasculature, decreased astrocyte hypertrophy, and microglial activation in the hippocampus [27].

Resveratrol showed protective effects against neurodegenerative diseases by enhancing the secretion of neurotransmitters, increasing the production of new neurons, decreasing neuroinflammation and oxidative stress, reducing neuronal apoptosis, and promoting hippocampal neurogenesis [28, 29]. However, these results need to be confirmed at the clinical stage in further studies with a specific patient categorization to adapt the supplementation strategy.

2.5 Antiaging action

Resveratrol is a polyphenolic sirtuin activator (SIRT-1), the first step in the process of deacetylation of peroxisome proliferator-activated receptor-coactivator (PGC-1a), which further modulates the genomic transcription of genes involved in mitochondrial metabolism. Resveratrol through the signaling cascade may be a regulator of multiple metabolic processes by activating SITR-1, which is present in many tissues, such as muscles, pancreas, and adipose tissues [30]. Administration of resveratrol (500 mg/day) in healthy and overweight subjects resulted in higher gene expression and serum concentration of sirtuin-1 [31], confirming the preclinical findings. Sirtuins exhibit a broad spectrum of bioactivities, including antiaging and anti-inflammatory effects, inhibition of degenerative disorders, such as liver steatosis, as well as improvement of endothelial function. Resveratrol induces neuronal differentiation in murine neuroblastoma cells and the differentiation of monocytes to macrophages. Intragastric administration or resveratrol causes activation of cardiac stem cells, an increase of capillary density, and reduction of apoptosis of cardiomyocytes, which may be beneficial in myocardial regeneration after acute myocardial infarction. Furthermore, by reducing the expression of perilipin 5, resveratrol accelerates lipid hydrolysis in brown adipose tissue, which may cause a decrease in weight and myocardial steatosis of heart tissue [32]. Supplementation with 0.04% resveratrol for 6 months in aging mice also reduces fatigue and enhances skeletal muscle function. Moreover, a daily dose of 500 mg of resveratrol relieves joint pain and stimulates the daily activity of patients with knee osteoarthritis [33]. Farrokhi et al. [34] demonstrated that 120 μM resveratrol reduced the production of matrix metalloproteinase 9, involved in atherosclerosis etiology.

Moreover, supplementation may influence DNA methylation and histone modification, pertinent in the context of obesity and energy metabolism. Histones' posttranscriptional modifications may be modulated by resveratrol. For instance, it influences histone deacetylation *via* sirtuins, and sirtuins activated by resveratrol can deacetylate sites on PGC1a [35].

Resveratrol may modulate different aspects of aging and tissue maintenance process through SIRT-1 signaling pathways from histone modification, DNA methylation, joint degenerative process, cardiac stem cells regulation, and anti-inflammatory pathways. However, these promising findings of mechanisms of action in aging-related pathologies need to be confirmed in large clinical studies to build new nutritional strategies for aging focused on prevention.

2.6 Action of resveratrol on gut microbiota

Upon ingestion, resveratrol migrates through the gastrointestinal tract. Approximately 70% of the resveratrol intake is absorbed. During digestion and absorption, resveratrol binds to several nutrients, such as proteins, and the solubility of these will influence resveratrol absorption or excretion [36]. About 70–75% may enter the enterocyte, while the remaining 25% is directly excreted. Once inside the cell, 60% is glucuronidated and 13.5% is sulfated. These conjugates partially return to the intestine, leaving 17% glucuronides and 1.5% sulfates in the bloodstream [35]. The gut microbiota actively participates in resveratrol metabolism by increasing its availability from resveratrol precursors and producing resveratrol derivatives. A fraction is absorbed in the colon, where they are metabolized by the gut microbiota into low molecular weight phenolic compounds to be then transported to the liver, where they undergo further metabolizations: leading to the production of dihydroresveratrol, 3,4′- dihydroxy-trans-stilbene, and 3,4′-dihydroxybibenzyl, as main known metabolites to date. The bioactivity of resveratrol metabolites may be higher for some than resveratrol itself, and the antioxidant and anti-inflammatory of dihydroresveratrol was detected both *in vitro* and *in vivo* [30]. The exact bioactivities of resveratrol derivatives are not exactly well known.

It has been reported that resveratrol may also modulate gut microbial composition, while microbiota also regulates resveratrol biotransformation. Resveratrol is known to modulate the composition of the gut microbiota with a decrease in opportunistic pathogenic bacteria *in vivo*. Qiao et al. demonstrated that resveratrol supplementation at the daily dose of 200 mg/kg/d for 12 weeks promotes a higher Bacteroidetes-to-firmicutes ratio in western-diet-fed mice. In addition, the number of lactobacillus and Bifidobacterium was significantly increased in resveratrol-fed animals [37]. They are closely linked with redox signaling in mucosal epithelial cells, which plays a critical role in maintaining gut homeostasis. Moreover, Enterococcus faecalis, a pathogenic bacterium, was significantly decreased in resveratrol-fed mice. Similarly, recent evidence suggests that the relative abundance of Bacteroides, lactobacillus, Bfidobacterium, and akkermansia is increased with resveratrol supplementation. These effects on the modulation of the gut flora may be associated with anti-obesity effect. Resveratrol administration leads to an increase in the number of lactobacillus species and a decrease in the number of E. faecalis and E. coli in high-fat diet (HFD) mice. Both E. faecalis and E. coli are positively correlated with colonic ROS and MDA levels. Resveratrol also inhibits the growth of Bacteroides and Desulfovibrionaceae spp.; enhancing the proportion of blautia and dorea in the lachnospiraceae family, participating in the improvement of lipid and glycemic profile in HFD-rodent model of metabolic alterations and obesity. This was confirmed in another study. In HFD mice, resveratrol supplementation modulated the microbiota composition, suggesting a prebiotic action. The microbiota changes were characterized by a decreased abundance of pathogenic bacteria, such as desulfovibrio, lachnospiraceae_NK4A316_group, and alistipes, as well as an increased abundance of short-chain fatty acid (SCFA)-producing bacteria, such as allobaculum, Bacteroides, and blautia. Moreover, transplantation of the HFD resv-microbiota into HFD group triggers a reduction in body weight, chronic inflammation, and improved liver steatosis and hepatic lipid metabolism [38]. Resveratrol treatment for 25 days in DSS-colitis rat model leads to beneficial effects on the colon, including the modulation of the inflammation-associated genes, colonic mucosa architecture normalization, and the modulation of NF-kB pathway. Resveratrol administration can also rebalance normal intestinal microbiota in bacterial composition.

These data suggest a prebiotic activity of resveratrol, which modifies the variability and composition of the intestinal microbiota, with a decrease in the firmicutes/Bacteroidetes ratio, which is increased in obese patients [39].

Resveratrol may reduce chronic inflammation through changes in the gut microbiota. Resveratrol and its microbial metabolites may inhibit the increased levels of ROS, activate Nrf2 signaling, and improve oxidative stress associated with chronic inflammatory conditions. They also protect epithelial barrier function and help decrease the activation of NF-κB and intestinal inflammation. Resveratrol may also modulate gut microbiota composition by enhancing beneficial endogenous strains, such as bifidobacterial or lactobacillus, and inhibit harmful pathogens [40].

2.7 Cardiometabolic action of resveratrol

Oral administration of resveratrol activates SIRT-1 and its targets, such as nuclear factor kappa B (NF-kB) and (PGC-1a) in mammalian tissues. PGC1a, a key regulator of energy metabolism, leads to decreased glycolysis in muscle and the liver, and increased lipid catabolism. As a consequence, it influences both glucose metabolism and lipid metabolism, inhibiting their accumulation. Resveratrol promoted SIRT-1 and also SIRT-5, which are involved in cellular energy homeostasis and cellular longevity [41]. Its consumption improves insulin secretion, decreases insulin resistance by protecting pancreatic beta cells from oxidative stress and by improving insulin metabolism. Furthermore, resveratorl consumption is also associated with reduction in fasting blood glycemia and Hb1ac. Resveratrol activates AMPK, which upregulates insulin receptor substrate-1 as part of insulin signaling modulation. Resveratrol activated AMPK-a and promoted mitochondrial biogenesis in the skeletal muscle of diet-induced insulin-resistant rodents [42, 43]. Resveratrol reduces the expression of adiponectin, which regulates insulin sensitivity [44–46]. Franco et al., (2014) demonstrated that in a rodent model programmed to be at risk of obesity and leptin resistance by early weaning, resveratrol suppressed leptin resistance, which prevents body weight gain, hyperphagia hyperglycemia, insulin resistance and visceral obesity in adult rats. In tissues, where SIRT-1 is present, resveratrol controls the insulin responses of target cells [47]. In the liver, SIRT-1 acts on gluconeogenesis. Therefore, resveratrol is considered to mimic the effects of a low-calorie diet, which improves cell turnover by slowing down the aging process [48].

In adipose tissue, resveratrol inhibits the process of the formation and accumulation of fat in the white adipose tissue. Moreover, resveratrol has been demonstrated to decrease body fat accumulation and leptin messenger ribonucleic acid (mRNA) levels and improve insulin sensitivity [49]. Resveratrol-induced reduction in fat mass is due to the activation of lipolysis through the adipose triglyceride lipase and the inhibition of de novo lipogenesis with the modulation of lipogenic enzymes and sterol regulatory element-binding protein-1c [36]. Resveratrol stimulates the production of brown adipose tissue and activates its metabolism by enhancing AMPK-α1 signaling in HFD mice. Moreover, activation of AMPK and SIRT-1 signaling with resveratrol, induces the browning of WAT. Resveratrol supplementation triggers SIRT-1 induced activation of PPAR signaling and PGC-1α in adipocytes, leading to fat browning [41, 50]. Resveratrol treatment has been demonstrated to decrease lipogenesis and increase lipolysis; thus, having an anti-obesity effect. It has also been shown to increase the capacity of thermogenesis in brown adipose tissue. Resveratrol treatment inhibited preadipocyte proliferation, adipogenic differentiation, and inflammatory cytokines production in a SIRT1-dependent manner.

Resveratrol may activate SIRT-1 and SIRT-3, and further improve mitochondrial metabolism, which in turn decreases ROS production, increases FA oxidation, and inhibits the damage of fatty acid synthase (FAS). As a consequence, resveratrol increases mitochondrial biogenesis and decreases mitochondrial uncoupling protein-2 (UCP-2) expression by activating SIRT-1 in β-cells [51].

Resveratrol may also improve some risk factors of cardiovascular health. The administration of resveratrol results in a reduced formation of trimethylamine-N-oxide (TMAO), a metabolite of carnitine and choline, considered as a risk factor for heart attack and stroke as it activates platelet activity, enhancing the risk of thrombosis. IL-1, IL-6, C-reactive protein, and the transcriptional activity of nuclear factor kappa B (NF-kB), which regulate inflammatory processes and immune responses, are reduced in patients with cardiovascular diseases, showing improvements in hypertension and ischemic heart disease risk [52]. Moreover, resveratrol treatment significantly lowered aorta media thickness, inflammation, fibrosis, and oxidative stress in aged male C57BL/6 mice compared to the control group, protecting against arterial aging by modulating the activity of the renin-angiotensin system [41]. Resveratrol could reduce superoxide generation, enhance NO level, and improve oxidative stress; thus, protecting against aging-associated vascular diseases [53, 54].

Other animal studies, mainly conducted in rats, have shown a reduction of abdominal fat, lipoprotein lipase, and ACC activities after treatment with resveratrol the anti-obesity effect of resveratrol is partly due to alteration in the gut microbiome and its related consequences [55].

Various different studies have reported that resveratrol has a high value to decrease insulin resistance, and improve glucose, lipid homeostasis, and cardiometabolic risk [35, 51, 56] through sirtuine signaling pathways, antioxidant, anti-inflammatory, and gut microbiota modulation (composition and bioactivities).

3. Resveratrol consumption is associated with promising health benefits: review of clinical data

Resveratrol is associated with many preclinical benefits demonstrated in a wide range of health axis. At the clinical evidence stage, the strength of evidence differs depending on number of studies available, heterogeneity in trial design and methodology, duration of studies, and population profile. This part will summarize the clinical evidence available in diabetes, obesity, cardiovascular health, metabolic health, and women health, based on meta-analysis and Randomized Controlled Trials (RCT) (**Figure 3**).

3.1 Diabetes

Diabetes is a silent disease that is associated with inappropriate eating habits and lifestyles. By 2045 more than 11% of the world population would be diagnosed. Diabetes is an important risk factor for mortality since it is associated with years of life lost. In addition to elevated fasting glycemia, diabetic patients often have metabolic syndrome comorbidities, such as obesity, hypertension, and dyslipidemia, all of which enhance the risk of diabetic complications, especially cardiovascular diseases. Moreover, clinical data also suggested that 30–40% of patients will have at least one complication about 10 years after the onset of diabetes, suggesting the importance of a new nutritional approach and complementary approach.

A first meta-analysis included randomized clinical trials with humans that evaluated the effects of resveratrol supplementation, compared to placebo, in type 2 diabetes treatment or prevention [57]. 24 RCT were included. Results showed that resveratrol supplementation had no significant effect on fasting blood glucose compared to placebo. However, results showed that there was a significant reduction in insulin resistance in individuals treated with resveratrol. Resveratrol also showed a

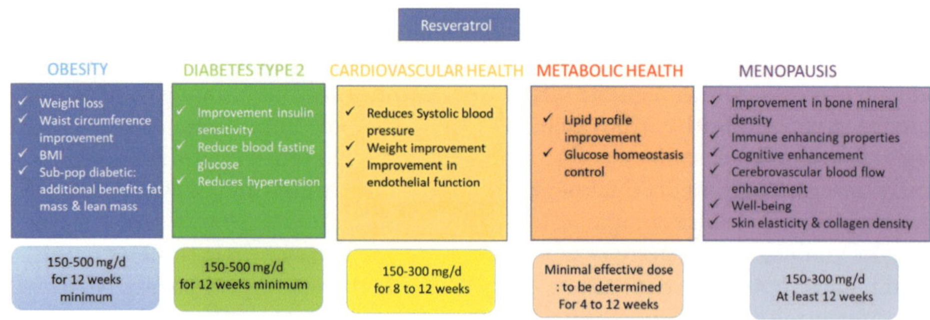

Figure 3.
Main clinical benefits reported by resveratrol and associated conditions of use.

significant reduction in Hb1ac after a duration of use of more than 8 weeks. A previous meta-analysis that included only individuals with diabetes showed benefits from resveratrol supplementation on diabetes parameters like fasting blood glucose and insulin resistance [58].

A third meta-analysis included 19 studies involving 1151 patients with type 2 diabetes, including 584 patients treated with resveratrol and 567 patients who received a placebo [59] gives interesting additional insights. Compared with the control data group, large doses of resveratrol (≥1000 mg) reduced fasting blood glucose levels. Additionally, resveratrol reduced systolic blood pressure and diastolic blood pressure in patients with type 2 diabetes but did not improve waist circumference triglyceride levels or high-density lipoprotein cholesterol levels in patients with type 2 diabetes. A daily dose of resveratrol ranging from 5 mg to 5 g for at least 12 months improves glycemia and insulin sensitivity in diabetic patients These meta-analysis pointed out promising results in DT2 patients supplemented with resveratrol for at least 8 to 12 weeks. The minimal effective dose needs to be determined for each DT2 patient profile, taking into account medical history and/or comorbidities.

3.2 Obesity

The first meta-analysis on 7 RCT on overweight and obese (BMI > 25) with or without comorbidities linked to obesity and daily doses ranging from 40 to 3000 mg/day [60] shows that the majority of studies were carried out with a supplementation superior to 150 mg/day for at least 4 weeks. A higher daily dose of resveratrol ranging from 400 to 600 mg was associated with improvements in insulin sensitivity, lipid profile, metabolic flexibility, total antioxidant capacity, increase in energy expenditure and reduction of ectopic accumulation of fat. Moreover, a lower dosage at 150 mg/day for 30 days significantly decreased the metabolic rate of sleep in obese patients without increaseing the energy expenditure. There was also an increase in 24 h respiratory quotient values, mainly during the day and postprandial period, suggesting an improvement in metabolic efficiency. After 4 weeks of supplementation at a daily dose of 150 mg in patients with obesity, there was an increase in SIRT-1 and an improvement in insulin sensitivity by lowering insulin concentration and HOMA-IR, compared to placebo.

A second meta-analysis included 28 randomized controlled trials, which were included on obese adults, healthy adults, and chronic inflammatory diseases including NAFLD, diabetes, and metabolic syndrome mainly [61]. Pooled effect sizes suggested a significant effect of resveratrol administration on weight, BMI, and waist circumference. No significant effect of resveratrol supplementation on fat mass was found. Subgroup analysis revealed a significant reduction in body weight and BMI for daily dosage <500 mg, those with long-term interventions (≥3 month), and performed on people with obesity.

A third meta-analysis on RCT was conducted to summarize the effect of resveratrol intake on weight loss [62]. Out of 831 reports, 36 RCTs were eligible for inclusion in our meta-analysis. The pooled results, using a random-effects model showed that resveratrol supplementation significantly decreased body weight, BMI, and waist circumference, which confirmed the results of Mousavi et al. The impact on weight loss was significant in sub-group analysis for obese and diabetic people. Overall, resveratrol intake significantly reduced weight, BMI, WC, and fat mass, and significantly increased lean mass, but did not affect leptin and adiponectin levels.

3.3 Cardiovascular health

In vitro and in vivo studies demonstrated that resvereatrol has antiatherogenic, antihypertensive properties. It also promotes vasodilatation through the increase of NO production. Moreover, resveratrol reduces vascular oxidative stress, prevents vascular remodeling and reduces arterial stiffness. In addition, resveratrol also inhibits immune cell infiltration into the vascular wall and mitigates vascular inflammation [63]. Two recent meta-analyses assessed the potential clinical benefits on cardiovascular health.

The first meta-analysis on 17 randomized clinical studies on 681 subjects [64]. The daily dose ranged from 75 to 3000 mg/day and the duration was from 4 weeks to 6 months. No significant effect was observed on BP, SBP, or DBP. A significant weight mean difference in the diabetic population was observed. A positive association between SBP and BMI was significant. The cardiovascular factors were improved, especially at higher doses than 300 mg/day in the diabetic population. Another meta-analysis, including 6 RCT, comprising a total of 247 subjects were selected. Resveratrol consumption may not significantly reduce SBP and DBP. Subgroup analyses indicated that higher-dose of resveratrol consumption (>150 mg/d) significantly reduces SBP, whereas the lower dose of resveratrol did not show a significant lowering effect on SBP. The meta-regression analyses did not indicate the dose effects of resveratrol on SBP or DBP [65].

It could be promising regarding the preliminary results observed in clinical studies but additional clinical studies for atherosclerosis, hypertension, stroke, and myocardial infarction are needed to estimate the minimal effective dose, and duration of supplementation for each target population [54]. The minimal effective dose for SBP regulation in hypertension may be >150 mg/day to be confirmed in additional clinical studies on hypertensive subjects.

3.4 Metabolic health

Chronic diseases are generally slow-progressing and long-duration diseases. They are also named noncommunicable diseases. Based on the definition of World Health Organization (WHO), there are four major noncommunicable diseases, including cardiovascular diseases, cancers, diabetes, and chronic respiratory diseases (World Health Organization, 2013), representing a leading cause of death.

A first meta-analysis reviewed the effect of supplementation on noncommunicable disease risk factors, such as fasted glycemia, lipid profile, and BP [66]. Out of the total, 29 RCTs with 1069 participants were included. The dose of resveratrol supplementation ranged from 10 to 3000 mg, and the duration of intervention lasted from 4 weeks to 12 months. Resveratrol supplementation significantly reduced blood fasting glucose, total cholesterol, and CRP. Resveratrol supplementation is associated with significant reductions in SBP and DBP in DT2 patients. Subgroup analysis demonstrated that the clinical studies with resveratrol intervention superior to 3 months significantly reduced the LDL-cholesterol, DBP, and HbA1c values. However, no significant improvement was found in HDL-C TG, and insulin resistance score (HOMA-IR) after resveratrol supplementation.

A second meta-analysis was performed on 21 RCT, including NAFLD, diabetic patients, healthy adults, and adults with dyslipidemia [67]. The daily doses range from 10 to 500 mg/day and the duration of supplementation is from 4 to 12 weeks. The results have shown that it may significantly reduce total cholesterol, but no significant effects on LDL-C, HDL-C, and TG were observed. The differences between both meta-analyses may vary in lipid profile, depending on the type of population selected in the analysis.

Resveratrol treatment has also demonstrated clinical benefits on glucose and lipid metabolism confirmed in a meta-analysis. Study population, resveratrol source, and daily dose have varied greatly, potentially explaining inconsistent findings. Improvements were mainly observed in endothelial function, systolic blood pressure, as well as markers of oxidative stress and chronic inflammation in several studies [68]. Resveratrol supplementation significantly decreased body weight, BMI, and waist circumference based on several recent meta-analyses. Further clinical studies are needed to optimize and adapt the conditions of use (dose, duration) for specific patients' profile (diabetes, metabolic health, obesity, and cardiovascular health) but promising clinical evidence shows the potential of resveratrol for cardiometabolic health management as a complementary approach to medical usual care.

3.5 Cognitive health

The societal impact of age-related cognitive decline is likely to be compounded by the global aging population, with a predicted doubling in the number of persons aged >60 years by 2050. Resveratrol reduces inflammatory cytokine release, improves mitochondrial energetic function, and improves A*b*-peptide clearance by activating SIRT-1 and AMPK [69]. Some positive findings on depression rodent models as a potential mood-enhancing agent are promising [70]. A meta-analysis was also conducted to determine the treatment effect on the following cognitive domains and mental processes: processing speed, number facility, memory, and mood [69]. In total, 10 studies were included on 372 individuals. Three studies found resveratrol supplementation significantly improved some measures of cognitive performance, two reported mixed findings, and five found no effect. When data were pooled, resveratrol supplementation had a significant effect on delayed recognition and negative mood. The results of this review indicate that resveratrol supplementation might improve select measures of cognitive performance. The dose of resveratrol used in the included studies ranged from 75–500 mg with no clear dose-dependent effect, suggesting that the differences in trial results may potentially not be due to the dosage used. Resveratrol shows promise as a complementary treatment in neuroprotection agents by improving cognitive function and reducing AD pathologies, such as A*b*. These benefits seem to be driven by improvements in brain metabolism through the regulation of ROS production, inflammation, and by preventing mitochondrial dysfunction. The benefits of resveratrol on brain health highlight that alteration in brain metabolism drive the future potential severity of the cognitive decline. The impact of inflammation and mitochondrial dysfunction on neuronal health explains to the promise on cognition as a neuroprotective agent [71, 72]. Further clinical studies are needed in this field of research due to promising preliminary findings.

3.6 Women's health

Menopausal women have an increased risk of developing NCDs due to hormonal dysregulation and the ongoing aging process. Menopause is also linked to various daily discomfort due to estrogen deficit and hormonal changes, such as vasomotor symptoms (diurnal hot flushes and night sweats), muscular and joint weakness or pain, sleep disorders, mood variations, vaginal dryness, skin dryness, and wrinkles appearance, which impacts the quality of life of women, body image, and their social interaction. The prevalence of dementia is from 14–32% higher for women than for men over 65 years old; by the age of 80, women account for 63% of dementia sufferers worldwide and this difference is expected to become more pronounced [73].

A pilot study in overweight and obese postmenopausal women with high body mass index (BMI ≥ 25 kg/m2) to determine the clinical effect of resveratrol on systemic sex steroid hormones [74]. Forty subjects initiated the resveratrol intervention (1 g daily for 12 weeks). Resveratrol intervention triggers a 10% increase in the concentrations of sex steroid hormone binding globulin (SHBG) notably. Resveratrol intervention resulted in 73% increase in urinary 2-hydroxyestrone (2-OHE1) levels leading to a favorable change in the urinary 2-OHE1/16α-OHE1 ratio.

Lymphocytes from 13 healthy menopausal women were isolated and then cocultured with hTERT-HME1, a breast cell line with a precancerous phenotype. The results demonstrated that resveratrol treated lymphocytes significantly increased TNF-a production, the formation of immune synapses, and the target cell lysis. No significant effect was observed in the lymphocyte total antioxidant capacity. These results demonstrate that resveratrol may stimulate immune surveillance in menopausal women by increasing the cytotoxic activity of lymphocytes [75].

A first meta-analysis analyzed the effect of resveratrol on bone health, and relevant to women's health [76]. Pooling six RCTs (eight treatment arms with 264 subjects) together. The dose of resveratrol ranged from 150 to 1500 milligrams per day. The duration of intervention also varied from 6 to 24 weeks, and no significant reduction of serum calcium, osteocalcin, C-terminal telopeptide of type I collagen, and procollagen I N-terminal propeptide values after resveratrol supplementation over placebo treatment. However, a significant increase in serum alkaline phosphatase (ALP) and bone alkaline phosphatase (BAP) values was observed after resveratrol treatment relative to placebo. The findings of this meta-analysis indicate that resveratrol supplementation increased some key bone biomarkers, such as ALP and BAP. This was confirmed in another large RCT in chronic use. The resveratrol for healthy aging in women (RESHAW) trial was a 24-month randomized, double-blind, placebo-controlled, and two-period crossover intervention carried out to assess the effects of resveratrol supplementation (75 mg twice daily) on cognition, cerebrovascular function, bone health, and cardiometabolic markers in 129 postmenopausal women [77]. After 12 months of supplementation, there were positive effects on bone density measured in the lumbar spine and neck of the femur, which was accompanied by a 7.24% reduction in C-terminal telopeptide type-1 collagen levels, a bone resorption marker, and compared with placebo. The increase in bone mineral density in the femoral neck resulted in a reduction in the 10-year probability of major and hip fracture risk. In the crossover comparison, the benefit of resveratrol over placebo on lumbar spine BMD was enhanced in those who regularly supplemented with both vitamin D and calcium compared with the calcium-only group [78]. The chronic supplementation of resveratrol combined with vitamin D and calcium may be interesting as a prevention strategy for bone weakness, fractures, and falls in menopausal women.

Eighty postmenopausal women aged 45–85 years were randomized to consume trans-resveratrol at a daily dose of 150 mg or placebo for 14 weeks. The effects of resveratrol on cognitive performance, cerebral blood flow velocity, and pulsatility index (a measure of arterial stiffness) in the middle cerebral artery and cerebrovascular responsiveness (CVR) were measured. Mood questionnaires were also administered. Resveratrol displayed 17% increases in CVR to both hypercapnic and cognitive stimuli compared to placebo group. Significant improvements were also observed in mental performance in the domain of verbal memory and in overall cognitive performance, which correlated with the increase in CVR. Following resveratrol supplementation, anxiety was significantly reduced. No significant changes were observed in other components of the POMS or in depressive symptoms [79].

Another 14-week randomized, double-blind, placebo-controlled clinical trial with resveratrol (75 mg, twice daily) was carried out in 80 healthy postmenopausal women [77]. Pain, menopausal symptoms, sleep quality, depressive symptoms, mood, and quality of life were assessed by SF-36 questionnaire at baseline and end of treatment. Compared with the placebo treatment, there was a significant reduction in pain and an improvement in total well-being after resveratrol supplementation. Benefits in quality of life are correlated with improvements in cerebrovascular function.

A 24-month randomized, placebo-controlled study was carried out in 125 postmenopausal women, aged 45–85 years, who consume 75 mg of resveratrol and a placebo twice daily for 12 months for each treatment in a cross-over design [79]. Compared to placebo, resveratrol supplementation resulted in a significant 33% improvement in overall cognitive performance. Women >65 years of age showed a relative improvement in verbal memory with resveratrol compared to those younger than 65 years. Furthermore, resveratrol improved secondary outcomes, including resting mean CBFV (cerebral blood flow velocity), fasting insulin, and insulin resistance index (HOMA-IR); Regular supplementation with low-dose resveratrol may enhance cognition, cerebrovascular function, and insulin sensitivity in postmenopausal women, to be confirmed in additional studies.

Formulations with resveratrol may also be useful for skin health maintenance during menopause. It may enhance the proliferation of fibroblasts, contributing to the increase in collagen III production. Resveratrol can bind ERα and Erβ estrogen receptors, participating in the stimulation of collagen types I and II production. RESV-mediated effects on keratinocyte senescence and proliferation are regulated by the AMPK FOXO3 pathway besides than by SIRT-1 [80]. Moreover, resveratrol exerts antioxidant action and may protect cells against oxidative stress associated with the deleterious action of free radicals and UV radiation on the skin by reducing the expression of AP-1 and NF-kB factors. Resveratrol may downregulate the process of photoaging of the skin [81]. Resveratrol has been demonstrated to act on cellular signaling mechanisms related to UV-mediated photoaging, including MAP kinases, nuclear factor kappa B (NF-kB), and matrix metalloproteinases [82]. Additionally, it has antiproliferative, anti-angiogenic, anti-inflammatory, antioxidant, and antimicrobial properties for cosmetic use in topical use or nutricosmetic for improving skin metabolism especially during menopause when hormonal disbalance leads to skin metabolism alterations. Resveratrol, with its structural similarity with diethylstilbestrol, a synthetic estrogen, may be considered a phytoestrogen. Indeed, resveratrol may activate the transcription of estrogen-responsive reporter genes and its action was inhibited by specific estrogen antagonists. This estrogen like effect may increase skin moisturization, skin elasticity, and thickness, as well as reducing skin wrinkles size and increase skin collagen content and the level of vascularization [83].

4. Conclusion

Resveratrol has been clinically tested in a wide range of health axis from cardiometabolic health, including diabetes, obesity, cardiovascular risk factors, neurocognitive health, and women's health with identified mechanisms of action implying various cellular pathways. Resveratrol is naturally occurring in wine but innovations also produce it as a purified substance from a specific patented chemical process. A novel food application has been granted for resveratrol by EFSA in Europe for use of 99% trans-resveratrol, and the intended intake level of 150 mg/day for adults does not raise safety concerns to be used in food supplements (EFSA Journal 2016;14(1):4368). The bioavailability of resveratrol may be enhanced through the use of a specific production process or the adjunction of quercetin, which is believed to inhibit the sulfation of resveratrol in the body and increase its bioavailability. A food supplement represents a concentrated source of actives to support physiological functions of the body, resveratrol may be used in food supplements targeting women's health, cognitive health, and metabolic health, which mainly help in transient discomfort and support the natural functions in healthy adults, especially when the body is subject to mental or physical stress, seasonal changes, aging or as an adjunct complementary approach in metabolic in glycemic control, lipid profile, weight management, or cardiovascular risk management.

FSMP are foods for specific medical purposes regulated by European regulatory texts n° 609/2013 and regulation EC 2016/128. For specific pathologies, especially targeting aging, malnutrition, and chronic inflammatory diseases (neurodegenerative disease, NAFLD, diabetes, and IBD). Resveratrol may also be used to modulate physiological signaling pathways involving oxidative stress reduction, anti-inflammatory action, SIRT-1 modulation, and neuroprotective action notably. As a cosmetic ingredient to be used in topical use or in food supplements in nutricosmetics, resveratrol has promising beneficial effects on skin health. Resveratrol may be considered a valuable ingredient in a nutritional complementary approach for various health axis to be confirmed in further clinical and to be considered by healthcare practitioners, dieticians, and pharmacists as a prevention or complementary approach in the personalized nutritional program.

Author details

Veronique Traynard
RNI Conseil, Angers, France

*Address all correspondence to: veronique.traynard@gmail.com

References

[1] Galiniak et al. Health benefits of resveratrol administration. Acta Biochimica Polonica. 2019;**66**(1):13-21

[2] Liu Y, He XQ, Huang X, Ding L, Xu L, Shen YT, et al. Resveratrol protects mouse oocytes from methylglyoxal-induced oxidative damage. PLoS One. 2013;**8**:e77960. DOI: 10.1371/journal.pone.0077960

[3] Liguori I, Russo G, Curcio F, Bulli G, Aran L, Della-Morte D, et al. Oxidative stress, aging, and diseases. Clinical Interventions in Aging. 2018;**13**:757-772. DOI: 10.2147/CIA.S158513

[4] Plauth A, Geikowski A, Cichon S, Wowro SJ, Liedgens L, Rousseau M, et al. Hormetic shifting of redox environment by pro-oxidative resveratrol protects cells against stress. Free Radical Biology & Medicine. 2016;**99**:608-622. DOI: 10.1016/j.freeradbiomed.2016.08.006

[5] Zhou R, Yi L, Ye X, Zeng X, Liu K, Qin Y, et al. Resveratrol ameliorates lipid droplet accumulation in liver through a SIRT1/ATF6-dependent mechanism. Cellular Physiology and Biochemistry. 2018;**51**:2397-2420. DOI: 10.1159/000495898

[6] Hussein MM, Mahfouz MK. Effect of resveratrol and rosuvastatin on experimental diabetic nephropathy in rats. Biomedicine & Pharmacotherapy. 2016;**82**:685-692. DOI: 10.1016/j.biopha.2016.06.004

[7] Corrêa MG, Absy S, Tenenbaum H, Ribeiro FV, Cirano FR, Casati MZ, et al. Resveratrol attenuates oxidative stress during experimental periodontitis in rats exposed to cigarette smoke inhalation. Journal of Periodontology Research. 2018;**54**:225-232. DOI: 10.1111/jre.12622

[8] Lin YT, Wu YC, Sun GC, Ho CY, Wong TY, Lin CH, et al. Effect of resveratrol on re- active oxygen species-induced cognitive impairment in rats with angiotensin II-induced early Alzheimer's disease. Journal of Clinical Medicine. 2018;7:329. DOI: 10.3390/jcm7100329

[9] Wang XL, Li T, Li JH, Miao SY, Xiao XZ. The effects of resveratrol on inflammation and oxidative stress in a rat model of chronic obstructive pulmonary disease. Molecules. 2017;**22**:1529. DOI: 10.3390/molecules22091529

[10] Ohtsu A, Shibutani Y, Seno K, Iwata H, Kuwayama T, Shirasuna K. Advanced glycation end products and lipopolysaccharidesstimulateinterleukin-6 secretion via the RAGE/TLR4-NF-κB-ROS pathways and resveratrol attenuates these inflammatory responses in mouse macrophages. Experimental and Therapeutic Medicine. 2017;**14**:4363-4370. DOI: 10.3892/etm.2017.5045

[11] Pinheiro DML, de Oliveira AHS, Coutinho LG, Fontes FL, de Medeiros Oliveira RK, Oliveira TT, et al. Resveratrol decreases the expression of genes involved in inflammation through transcriptional regulation. Free Radical Biology & Medicine. 2018;**130**:8-22. DOI: 10.1016/j.freeradbiomed.2018.10.432

[12] Malaguernera et al. Influence of resveratrol on the immune response. Nutrients. 2019;**11**:946

[13] Li C, Wu W, Jiao G, Chen Y, Liu H. Resveratrol attenuates inflammation and reduces matrix-metalloprotease expression by inducing autophagy via suppressing the Wnt/b-catenin signalling pathway in IL-1b-induced osteoarthritis

chondrocytes. RSC Advances. 2018;**8**:20202. DOI: 10.1039/c8ra00993g

[14] Yao W, Liu, et al. Anti-oxidant efects of resveratrol on mice with DSS-induced ulcerative colitis. Archives of Medical Research. 2010;**41**(4):288-294

[15] Misawa T, Saitoh T, Kozaki T, Park S, Takahama M, Akira S. Resveratrol inhibits the acetylated α-tubulin-mediated assembly of the NLRP3-inflammasome. International Immunology. 2015;**27**:425-434

[16] Yılmaz Z, Kalaz EB, Aydın AF, Olgaç V, Doğru-Abbasoğlu S, Uysal M, et al. The effect of resveratrol on glycation and oxidation products in plasma and liver of chronic methylglyoxal-treated rats. Pharmacological Reports. 2018;**70**:584-590. DOI: 10.1016/j.pharep.2017.12.005

[17] Ciddi V, Dodda D. Therapeutic potential of resveratrol in diabetic complications: In vitro and in vivo studies. Pharmacological Reports. 2014;**66**:799-803. DOI: 10.1016/j.pharep.2014.04.006

[18] Ma X, Sun Z, Liu Y, Jia Y, Zhang B, Zhang J. Resveratrol improves cognition and reduces oxidative stress in rats with vascular dementia. Neural Regeneration Research. 2013;**8**:2050-2059. DOI: 10.3969/j.issn.1673-5374.2013.22.004

[19] Corpas R, Griñán-Ferré C, Rodríguez-Farré E, Pallàs M, Sanfeliu C. Resveratrol induces brain resilience against Alzheimer neurodegeneration through proteostasis enhancement. Mol Neurobiol in press. 2018;**56**:1502-1516. DOI: 10.1007/s12035-018-1157-y

[20] Garrigue et al. Long-term administration of resveratrol at low doses improves neurocognitive performance as well as cerebral blood flow and modulates the inflammatory pathways in the brain. The Journal of Nutritional Biochemistry. 2021;**97**:108786. DOI: 10.1016/j.jnutbio.2021.108786

[21] Bonsack F, Alleyne CH Jr, Sukumari-Ramesh S. Resveratrol attenuates neurodegeneration and improves neurological outcomes after intracerebral hemorrhage in mice. Frontiers in Cellular Neuroscience. 2017;**11**:228. DOI: 10.3389/fncel.2017.00228

[22] Nalagoni CSR, Karnati PR. Protective effect of resveratrol against neuronal damage through oxidative stress in cerebral hemisphere of aluminum and fluoride treated rats. Interdisciplinary Toxicology. 2016;**9**:78-82. DOI: 10.1515/intox-2016-0009

[23] Lopez MS, Dempsey RJ, Vemuganti R. Resveratrol neuroprotection in stroke and traumatic CNS injury. Neurochemistry International. 2015;**89**:75-82. DOI: 10.1016/j.neuint.2015.08.009

[24] Torres-Perez RI, Tellez-Ballesteros, Ortiz-Lopez L, et al. Resveratrol enhances neuroplastic changes, including hippocampal neurogenesis, and memory in Balb/C mice at six months of age. PLoS One. 2015;**10**:21

[25] Zhao WF, Li F, Li, et al. Resveratrol improves learning and memory in normally aged mice through microRNA CREB pathway. Biochemical and Biophysical Research Communications. 2013;**435**(4):597-602

[26] Kodali VK, Parihar B, Hattiangady V, Mishra BS, Shetty AK. Resveratrol prevents age-related memory and mood dysfunction with increased hippocampal neurogenesis and microvasculature, and reduced glial activation. Scientific Reports. 2015;**5**:16

[27] Zhou et al. Effects and mechanisms of resveratrol on aging and age-related diseases. Oxidative Medicine and Cellular Longevity. 2021;**2021**:9932218, 15 pages. DOI: 10.1155/2021/9932218

[28] Grinan-Ferré et al. The pleiotropic neuroprotective effects of resveratrol in cognitive decline and Alzheimer's disease pathology: From antioxidant to epigenetic therapy. Aging Research reviews. 2021;**67**:191271

[29] Inchingolo et al. 2022, benefits and implications of resveratrol supplementation on microbiota modulations: A systematic review of the literature. International Journal of Molecular Sciences. 2022;**23**:4027

[30] Roggerio A, Strunz CMC, Pacanaro AP, Leal DP, Takada JY, Avakian SD, et al. Gene expression of sirtuin-1 and endogenous secretory receptor for advanced glycation end products in healthy and slightly overweight subjects after caloric restriction and resveratrol administration. Nutrients. 2018;**10**:937. DOI: 10.3390/nu10070937

[31] Ling L, Gu S, Cheng Y. Resveratrol activates endogenous cardiac stem cells and improves myocardial regeneration following acute myocardial infarction. Molecular Medicine Reports. 2017;**15**:1188-1194. DOI: 10.3892/mmr.2017.6143

[32] Hussain SA, Marouf BH, Ali ZS, Ahmmad RS. Efficacy and safety of co-administration of resveratrol with meloxicam in patients with knee osteoarthritis: A pilot interventional study. Clinical Interventions in Aging. 2018;**13**:1621-1630. DOI: 10.2147/CIA.S172758

[33] Farrokhi E, Ghatreh-Samani K, Salehi-Vanani N, Mahmoodi A. The effect of resveratrol on expression of matrix metalloproteinase 9 and its tissue inhibitors in vascular smooth muscle cells. ARYA Atheroscler. 2018;**14**:157-162. DOI: 10.22122/arya.v14i4.1484

[34] Springer & Moco. 2019, resveratrol and its human metabolites—Effects on metabolic health and obesity. Nutrients. 2019;**11**:143. DOI: 10.3390/nu11010143

[35] Chaplin et al. Resveratrol, metabolic syndrome, and gut microbiota. Nutrients. 2018;**10**:1651. DOI: 10.3390/nu10111651

[36] Qiao Y, Sun J, Xia S, Tang X, Shi Y, Le G. Effects of resveratrol on gut microbiota and fat storage in a mouse model with high-fat-induced obesity. Food & Function. 2014;**5**:1241-1249

[37] Wang et al. Targeting the gut microbiota with resveratrol: A demonstration of novel evidence for the management of hepatic steatosis. The Journal of Nutritional Biochemistry. 2020;**81**:108363

[38] Jasirwan et al. Correlation of gut Firmicutes/Bacteroidetes ratio with fibrosis and steatosis stratified by body mass index in patients with non-alcoholic fatty liver disease. Bioscience of Microbiota, Food and Health. 2021;**40**(1):50-58

[39] Hu et al. The bidirectional interactions between resveratrol and gut microbiota: An insight into oxidative stress and inflammatory bowel disease therapy. BioMed Research International. 2019;**2019**:5403761. 9 pages

[40] Kim MY, Kim JH, Lim et al. "The protective effect of resveratrol on vascular aging by modulation of the reninangiotensin system". Atherosclerosis. 2018;**270**:123-131

[41] Crandall JP, Oram V, Trandafirescu G, Reid M, Kishore P, Hawkins M, et al. Pilot study of resveratrol in older adults with impaired glucose tolerance. The Journals of Gerontology. Series A, Biological Sciences and Medical Sciences. 2012;**67**:1307-1312

[42] Knop FK, Konings E, Timmers S, Schrauwen P, Holst JJ, Blaak EE. Thirty days of resveratrol supplementation does not affect postprandial incretin hormone responses, but suppresses postprandial glucagon in obese subjects. Diabetes Medicine Journal of British Diabetic Association. 2013;**30**:1214-1218

[43] Zhang et al. Resveratrol ameliorates high-fat diet-induced insulin resistance and fatty acid oxidation via ATM-AMPK axis in skeletal muscle. European Review for Medical and Pharmacological Sciences. 2020;**23**:9117-9125

[44] Teng et al. 2020, resveratrol metabolites ameliorate insulin resistance in HepG2 hepatocytes by modulating IRS-1/AMPK. RSC Advances. 2018;**8**:36034-36042

[45] Mohammadi-Sartang et al. Resveratrol supplementation and plasma adipokines concentrations? A systematic review and meta-analysis of randomized controlled trials. Pharmacological Research. 2017;**117**:394-405. DOI: 10.1016/j.phrs.2017.01.012

[46] Franco JG et al. Resveratrol prevents hyperleptinemia and central leptin resistance in adult rats programmed by early weaning. Hormone Metab Res. 2014;**46**(10):728-735

[47] Frojdo S, Durand C, Pirola L. Metabolic effects of resveratrol in mammals—A link between improved insulin action and aging. Current Aging Science. 2008;**1**:145-151

[48] Eseberri I et al. Resveratrol metabolites modify adipokine expression and secretion in 3T3-L1 pre-adipocytes and mature adipocytes. PLoS One. 2013;**8**(5):1-8

[49] Mongioi et al. The role of resveratrol Administration in Human Obesity. International Journal of Molecular Sciences. 2021;**22**:4362. DOI: 10.3390/ijms22094362

[50] Huang et al. A review on the potential of resveratrol in prevention and therapy of diabetes and diabetic complications. Biomedicine & Pharmacotherapy. 2020;**125**:109767

[51] Wahab A, Gao K, Jia C, Zhang F, Tian G, Murtaza G, et al. Significance of resveratrol in clinical Management of Chronic Diseases. Molecular Journal of Synthesis Chemistry Natural Production Chemistry. 2017;**22**:1329

[52] Rajapakse A, Yepuri G, Carvas J, et al. Hyperactive S6K1 mediates oxidative stress and endothelial dysfunction in aging: Inhibition by resveratrol. PLoS One. 2011;**6**:16

[53] Bonnefont-Rousseleau. Resveratrol and cardiovascular diseases. Nutrients. 2016;**2016**(8):250. DOI: 10.3390/nu8050250

[54] Hou et al. The effects of resveratrol in the treatment of metabolic syndrome. International Journal of Molecular Sciences. 2019;**20**:535. DOI: 10.3390/ijms20030535

[55] Hoca M, et al. The role of resveratrol in diabetes and obesity associated with insulin resistance, Archives of Physiology and Biochemistry. 2021. DOI: 10.1080/13813455.2021.1893338

[56] Delpino & Figueiredo. Resveratrol supplementation and type 2 diabetes: A systematic review and meta-analysis.

Critical Reviews in Food Science and Nutrition. 2021;**62**:4465-4480. DOI: 10.1080/10408398.2021.1875980

[57] Gu et al. Effects of resveratrol on metabolic indicators in patients with type 2 diabetes: A systematic review and meta-analysis. Hindawi International Journal of Clinical Practice. 2022;**2022**:9734738. 19 pages. DOI: 10.1155/2022/9734738

[58] Zhu X, Wu C, Qiu S, Yuan X, Li L. Effects of resveratrol on glucose control and insulin sensitivity in subjects with type 2 diabetes: Systematic review and meta-analysis. Nutrition and Metabolism. 2017;**99**:1510-1519. DOI: 10.1186/s12986-017-0217-z

[59] Fraiz et al. 2021, can resveratrol modulate sirtuins in obesity and related diseases? A systematic review of randomized controlled trials. European Journal of Nutrition. 2021;**60**:2961-2977. DOI: 10.1007/s00394-021-02623-y

[60] Mousavi et al. Resveratrol supplementation significantly influences obesity measures: A systematic review and dose– Response meta analysis of randomized controlled trials. Obesity Reviews. 2018;**20**:487-498. DOI: 10.1111/obr.12775

[61] Tabrizi et al. The effects of resveratrol intake on weight loss: A systematic review and meta-analysis of randomized controlled trials. Critical Reviews in Food Science and Nutrition. 2018;**60**:375-390. DOI: 10.1080/10408398.2018.1529654

[62] Li et al. Resveratrol and vascular function. International Journal of Molecular Sciences. 2019;**20**:2155. DOI: 10.3390/ijms20092155

[63] Fogacci et al. Effect of resveratrol on blood pressure: A systematic review and meta-analysis of randomized, controlled, clinical trials. Critical Reviews in Food Science and Nutrition. 2018;**59**:1605-1618. DOI: 10.1080/10408398.2017.1422480

[64] Liu et al. Effect of resveratrol on blood pressure: A meta analysis of randomized controlled trials. Clinical Nutrition. 2015;**34**(1):27-34

[65] Guo et al. Effects of resveratrol supplementation on risk factors of non-communicable diseases: A metaanalysis of randomized controlled trials. Critical Reviews in Food Science and Nutrition. 2017;**58**:3016-3029. DOI: 10.1080/10408398.2017.1349076

[66] Haghighatdoost et al. Effect of resveratrol on lipid profile: An updated systematic review and meta-analysis on randomized clinical trials. Pharmacological Research. 2017;**129**:141-150. DOI: 10.1016/j.phrs.2017.12.033

[67] Pollack et al. Resveratrol: Therapeutic potential for improving Cardiometabolic health. American Journal of Hypertension. 2013;**26**(11):1260-1268

[68] Marx W, et al. Effect of resveratrol supplementation on cognitive performance and mood in adults: A systematic literature review and meta-analysis of randomized controlled trials. Nutrition Reviews VR. 2018;**76**(6):432-443

[69] Oliveira D et al. Molecular mechanisms underlying the anti-depressant effects of resveratrol: A review. Molecular Neurobiology. 2017;**55**:4543-4559. DOI: 10.1007/s12035-017-0680-6

[70] Yang et al. Resveratrol, metabolic dysregulation, and Alzheimer's disease: Considerations for Neurogenerative disease. International Journal of

Molecular Sciences. 2021;**22**:4628. DOI: 10.3390/ijms22094628

[71] Grignan-Ferré et al. The pleiotropic neuroprotective effects of resveratrol in cognitive decline and Alzheimer's disease pathology: From antioxidant to epigenetic therapy. Ageing Research Reviews. 2021;**67**:101271

[72] Monteleone et al. Symptoms of menopause - global prevalence, physiology and implications. Nature Reviews. Endocrinology. 2018;**14**(4):199-215

[73] Chow et al. A pilot clinical study of resveratrol in postmenopausal women with high body mass index: Effects on systemic sex steroid hormones. Journal of Translational Medicine. 2014;**12**:223

[74] Credico D et al. 2021, resveratrol enhances the cytotoxic activity of lymphocytes from menopausal women. Antioxidants. 1914;**2021**:10. DOI: 10.3390/antiox10121914

[75] Asis et al. Effects of resveratrol supplementation on bone biomarkers: A systematic review and meta-analysis. Annals. New York Academy of Sciences. 2019;**1457**:92-103. DOI: 10.1111/nyas.14226

[76] Wong et al. Resveratrol supplementation reduces pain experience by postmenopausal women. Menopause. 2017;**24**(8):916-922. DOI: 10.1097/GME.0000000000000861

[77] Evans et al. 2017, effects of resveratrol on cognitive performance, mood and cerebrovascular function in post-menopausal women; a 14-week randomised placebo-controlled intervention trial. Nutrients. 2017;**9**:27. DOI: 10.3390/nu9010027

[78] Wong et al. Regular supplementation with resveratrol improves bone mineral density in postmenopausal women: A randomized, placebo-controlled trial. Journal of Bone and Mineral Research. 2020;**35**(11):2121-2131

[79] Zaw et al. Long-term effects of resveratrol on cognition, cerebrovascular function and cardio-metabolic markers in postmenopausal women: A 24- month randomised, double-blind, placebo-controlled, crossover study. Clinical Nutrition. 2021;**40**:820-829. DOI: 10.1016/j.clnu.2020.08.025

[80] Wen et al. Role of resveratrol in regulating cutaneous functions. Evidence-Based Complementary and Alternative Medicine. 2020;**2020**. 20 pages:2416837. DOI: 10.1155/2020/2416837

[81] Ratz-Lyko A. Resveratrol as an active ingredient for cosmetic and dermatological applications: A review. Journal of Cosmetic and Laser Therapy. 2018;**21**:84-90. DOI: 10.1080/14764172.2018.1469767

[82] Baxter et al. Anti-aging properties of resveratrol: Review and report of a potent new antioxidant skin care formulation. Journal of Cosmetic Dermatology. 2008;**7**:2-7

[83] Chedea et al. Resveratrol from diet to topical usage. Food & Function. 2017;**8**:3879-3892. DOI: 10.1039/C7FO01086A

Chapter 5

Resveratrol Supplements Reduce the Risk of Aging-Related Cardiac Disease after Cardiorespiratory Fitness

Jia-Ping Wu, Zhu Xiaoning, Li Xiaoqing, Zhang Jie and Zhang Qian-Cheng

Abstract

Aging changes in the very elderly cardiac disease are associated with physiological and pathological changes, however, all observed changes in aging are associated with a deterioration of cardiorespiratory fitness function. For example, hypertension and cardiorespiratory disease make difficult distinctions between normal aging changes and the effects of underlying resveratrol supplements processes. Cardiorespiratory fitness-independent changes in resveratrol intake are still unclear. This review aimed to discuss whether the aging-associated cardiorespiratory fitness changes in the heart can be reversed by resveratrol supplements, and the mechanisms of cardiorespiratory fitness. Aging led to apoptosis and fibrosis-related protein expression increased, however, cardiorespiratory fitness had revered more functions. Resveratrol supplements in combination with cardiorespiratory fitness had a good enhanced mitochondrial function in aging including IL-6, STAT3, MEK5, and MEK1/ERK1 increased. Resveratrol supplements also induced survival signals and downregulation of apoptosis signaling in aging. Therefore, we suggest resveratrol has enhanced cardiorespiratory fitness to combine their function in repressed aging.

Keywords: physiological changes, aging, cardiorespiratory fitness, resveratrol supplements, left ventricular hypertrophy

1. Introduction

The global population is aging, the disease is younger and the influence of modern lifestyles, and because of climate change, global warming, and environmental pollution, etc., it has not been possible to effectively find a reasonable solution today. Technology, but it does also face the impact of modern diseases. It may be necessary to face the torture of the disease in advance, so the concept of health and advocating naturalness has gradually increased [1]. In terms of overall future business strategy, actively participate in chambers of commerce or related exhibitions, deliver related speeches, incorporate health-related cardiorespiratory fitness increases programs, shape and package soul figures, and expand virtual network access to business opportunities, public welfare, and cross-industry integration [2]. The fan club cardiorespiratory fitness operates and integrates resveratrol marketing through advertising and multimedia [3, 4]. It is expected to successfully introduce results into the online consumer resveratrol market, supplemented by online word-of-mouth marketing to expand online and offline marketing integration, increase market exposure, and find partners [5]. At the same time, network channels and physical channels are integrated. Through the integration of resveratrol intake and cardiorespiratory fitness increases strategies, cardiorespiratory fitness growth is promoted, and operations are gradually increased for humans [6]. Age-related cardiac disease is associated with numerous molecular and biochemical changes in the heart [7, 8]. These changes affect cardiorespiratory fitness protein function increases and cardiac morphology resulting in alterations in cell signaling [9]. The biochemical changes also affect the expression levels of mitochondrial membrane anti-apoptosis and apoptosis proteins [10]. Together, they achieve the original concept of saving people and saving the world, creating reasonable profits, and providing feedback to the people who have been supporting them for many years.

2. Resveratrol supplements

Resveratrol is a naturally occurring non-flavonoid polyphenol that exists in many plants, such as grapes, peanuts, and berries [11]. Natural resveratrol is a phytoalexin material to resist the invasion of bacteria produced. Resveratrol grape variety is a decisive factor in content [12]. Resveratrol is a polyphenol produced by plants in response to environmental stress (**Figure 1**). The trans-isomer of resveratrol is an effective anti-oxidant that scavenges free radicals [13]. Pharmacological studies suggest that therapeutic doses of resveratrol are non-toxic and well-tolerated by humans. Although present in small amounts in many plant-based foods, nutritional supplements of resveratrol are often produced from the extraction of resveratrol from the dried roots of *Polygonum cuspidatum*, which has also been used in traditional Asian medicine to treat cardiovascular disorders [14]. Resveratrol is rapidly and efficiently absorbed following oral administration, though its bioavailability is low due to its metabolism to sulfated and glucuronidation derivatives during first-pass metabolism. Most of the food resveratrol in the digestion process is an additional metal, that cannot be absorbed, only a very small number of parts can enter the circulatory system, and rely on the blood circulation of trans-resveratrol to achieve. According to reports, is a more effective absorption of the oral mucosa, and the oral jaw surface absorption efficiency of resveratrol than the stomach absorption is higher. Resveratrol is a compound Sirt 1 activation, thereby affecting the number of apoptosis, defense, and metabolic protein involved [15]. Aging is a complex process that is difficult to define. Physiological aging is generally defined to be a decline in body function that takes place in the absence of any discernible disease process. Thus, some reports reported resveratrol can induce free fatty acid release. Taking it, to gain lipid mobilization into the effects of resveratrol on regulated lipolytic activity in human adipocytes.

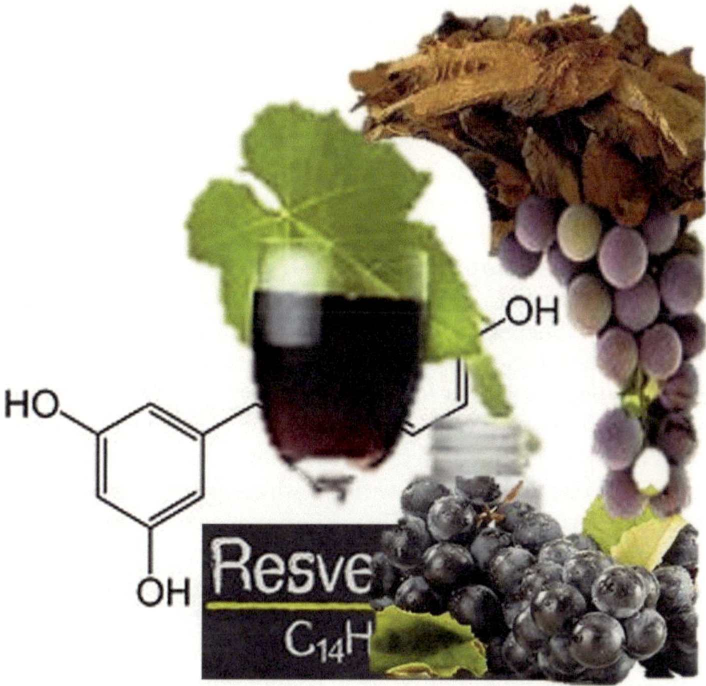

Figure 1.
Resveratrol supplements. Resveratrol is a natural compound found in red grape skin, peanuts, blueberries, and berries. Resveratrol supplements are a compound known as an antioxidant against environmental stresses and support in wine smaller doses could be quite beneficial for your health aging.

3. Resveratrol supplements and aging-related cardiac disease

Resveratrol supplementation has been reported to exert anti-inflammatory and anti-oxidant effects in humans. Resveratrol has also been shown to protect against cardiovascular aging diseases. Resveratrol supplementation intake is established regarding the major requirements for cardiorespiratory fitness and increased safety. Anti-aging effects of resveratrol supplementation improved physicochemical characterization and reversed diastolic pressure, cardiovascular remodeling, and cardiac functions [16]. Resveratrol supplements polyphenols have been reported for delaying aging and age-related cardiovascular diseases. Aging is malleable in many organisms which can induce senescence of cardiac fibrosis leading to a change in cardiac structure. Resveratrol was able to inhibit cardiac dysfunction and left ventricular hypertrophy (LVH) [17]. Resveratrol intake might be attenuated by aging-associated cardiovascular diseases, cardiac fibrosis, oxidative stress, inflammation, and contractility. Antioxidative may be affected the anti-aging process through resveratrol.

4. Resveratrol supplements and cardiorespiratory fitness increased

Cardiorespiratory fitness training improves the vasodilatory properties of the vasculature thereby optimizing O_2 transport throughout the body [18]. Regular Cardiorespiratory fitness also improves vascular function in association with the reduction of reactive oxygen species. In response to Cardiorespiratory fitness exercise, blood flow is markedly increased in contracting skeletal muscles and myocardium, but perfusion in other organs is only slightly enhanced or is even reduced (visceral organs). Moderate exercise has been evidenced responsible for O_2 transport unite of the body and the utilization of O_2 for the synthesis of ATP by cells, eventually. While moderate cardiorespiratory fitness accelerates O_2 entering the body via the lungs and functionally optimizes the organ systems to form an integrated unit to maintain or improve an active lifestyle [13]. Cardiorespiratory fitness is a physiological left ventricular hypertrophy adaptive response of the cardiomyocytes to physiological stresses in response to increased workload [19]. Cardiorespiratory fitness considers overlap exists between the mechanisms that control the pathological growth of the heart and the physiological growth of the heart. Increased cardiomyocyte cell size and protein synthesis are properties of both physiological and pathological left ventricular hypertrophy.

The specific purpose was to assess the involvement of resveratrol supplements and cardiorespiratory fitness increase. The effects of resveratrol alone and when combined with habitual cardiorespiratory fitness in aged-related heart disease. It was found in this review that supplementing with resveratrol during cardiorespiratory fitness could improve resveratrol intake performance, muscle strength, and whole-body oxidative metabolism (**Figure 2**). Since left ventricular hypertrophy is a positive adaptation to cardiorespiratory fitness, it appeared plausible that resveratrol treatment during cardiorespiratory fitness could block the physiologic growth of the myocardium and be deleterious [20]. Therefore, cardiorespiratory fitness increases may stimulate weight loss, glycemic control, insulin sensitivity, vagal tone, lean body mass, social support, vascular reactivity, and relaxation (**Figure 2**).

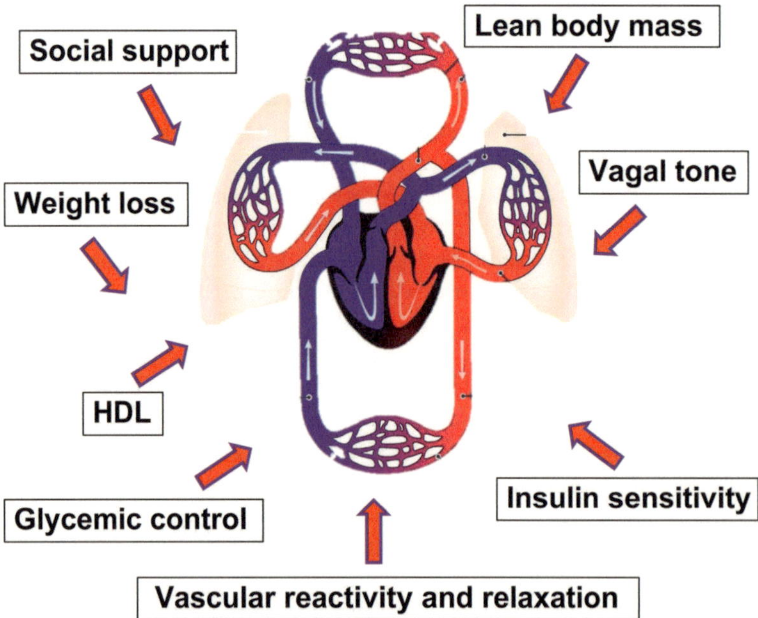

Figure 2.
High cardiorespiratory fitness. High cardiorespiratory fitness induced social support, weight loss, HDL, glycemic control, lean body mass, vagal tone, insulin sensitivity, vascular reactivity, and relaxation increases.

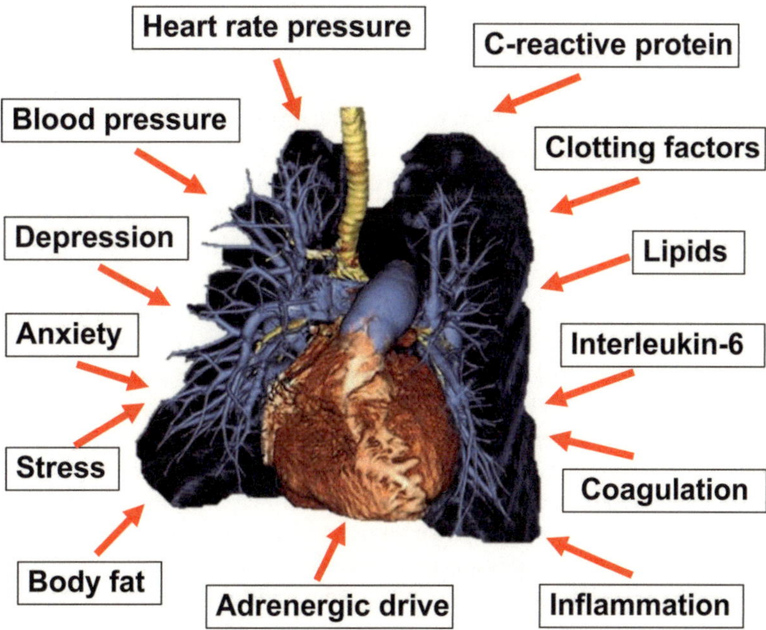

Figure 3.
Low cardiorespiratory fitness. Low cardiorespiratory fitness were resulted in heart rate pressure, blood pressure, depression, anxiety, stress, body fat, adrenergic drive, inflammation, coagulation, interleukin-6, lipids, clotting factors, and C-reactive protein decreases.

Lower cardiorespiratory fitness resulted in blood pressure, lipids, depression, anxiety, stress, body fat, inflammation, coagulation, clotting factors, heart rate pressure, adrenergic drive, C-reactive protein, and interleukin-6 (**Figure 3**). Thus, low cardiorespiratory fitness is associated with an increased risk for left ventricular hypertrophy and function in aging.

5. Resveratrol supplements in combination with cardiorespiratory fitness increased mechanisms

Cardiorespiratory fitness involves the combination of resveratrol supplementation emitted by aging and the cardiorespiratory fitness will reverse by resveratrol intake combination into the environment. Left ventricular pathological hypertrophy due to age was observed in old-age patients, which leads to left ventricular remodeling and loss of function [21]. In addition, IL6/MEK5/ERK5 regulates MEK1-ERK1/2 and JAK1/2-STAT1/3 to regulate cardiorespiratory fitness myocyte growth, apoptosis, and contractile function. IL-6 is a pro-inflammatory cytokine, that promotes tissue injury and cardiovascular pathologies. IL-6 after binding its gp130 receptor leads to cardiomyocyte hypertrophy, increased fibrosis, and heart failure. In contrast, the JAK/STAT pathway has been elucidated to late essential preconditioning of the cardiorespiratory fitness and cardiac hypertrophy, especially in pathological hypertrophy that proves heart function rupture [22]. The roles of TGF-β1 and MMPs (MMP2 and MMP9) in tissue remodeling are intertwined. However, the activities of MMPs are regulated by TIMPs. Moreover, TGF-β1 is induction through connective tissue growth factor to up-regulate pro-fibrotic proteins. These results demonstrated left ventricular hypertrophy in aging cardiorespiratory fitness. The Bcl-2 protein family plays a central role in the regulation of apoptosis. These proteins take part with antiapoptotic (Bcl-2, Bcl-xl) and pro-apoptotic members (Bax, Bad, Bak), whose reciprocal balance is fundamental in determining cell fate. The final execution phase, when it occurs, results in the activation of a family of proteases, the caspases, which participate in a cascade of events leading to the cleavage of a set of proteins, causing the disassembly of the cell. Until recently, little was known regarding the effects of cardiorespiratory fitness, resveratrol, and combining cardiorespiratory fitness and resveratrol supplementation on the physiological growth of aging cardiorespiratory fitness. While the aging-related mechanisms that define the distinct effects of cardiorespiratory fitness, resveratrol, and combining cardiorespiratory fitness and resveratrol intake on the myocardium in pathological and physiological situations remain to be defined, it is likely that the stimuli that promote pathological left ventricular hypertrophy (**Figure 4**). Left ventricular hypertrophy works through different signaling pathways than those that promote physiological left ventricular hypertrophy and resveratrol supplementation act to primarily inhibit those pathways that promote pathological left ventricular hypertrophy. Cardiorespiratory fitness aging is a human physiologic change that has slowly progressive structural changes and functional declines with age. Mitochondria may play an important role in apoptosis by releasing, Gαq, PKCβ, RhoA, p-JNK, p-P38, and p-ERK1 and antioxidative stress, SOD2, glutathione peroxidase, and catalase. While the increased hemodynamic load is the major factor in the development of pathological hypertrophy, alterations in molecular signaling pathways may also contribute to increased cardiomyocyte growth in autophagy in conjunction with and/or in the absence of increased afterload [23]. We aim to report the cardiorespiratory fitness changes of the elderly heart with resveratrol supplementary

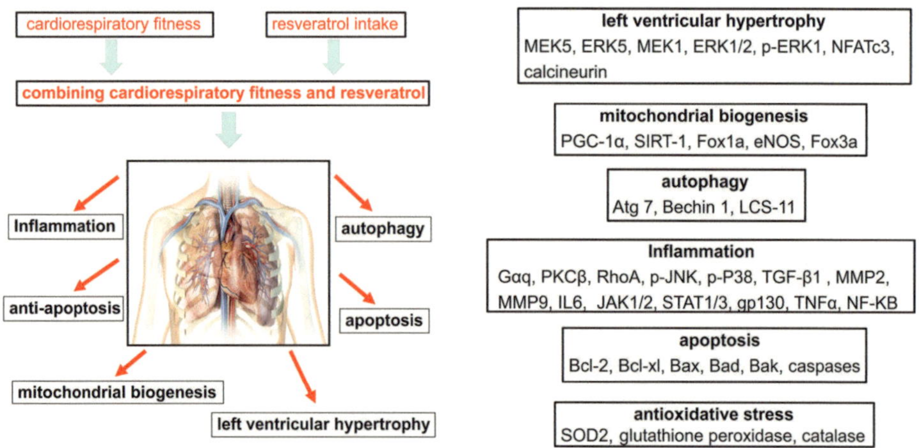

Figure 4.
The management consultant of cardiorespiratory fitness, resveratrol, and combining cardiorespiratory fitness and resveratrol. Combining cardiorespiratory fitness and resveratrol have benefits that are significant by mitochondrial biogenesis, left ventricular hypertrophy, autophagy, inflammation, apoptosis, and antioxidative stress.

supplementation which is expected for mitochondrial biogenesis and autophagy on normal aging cardiorespiratory fitness change. However, cardiorespiratory fitness increases with resveratrol, and combining exercise and resveratrol is associated with age-related pathology. Therefore, the effect of cardiorespiratory fitness increased by exercise with resveratrol, and combining cardiorespiratory fitness and resveratrol in aged hearts is interesting to be revealed mitochondrial biogenesis and autophagy. Mitochondrial biogenesis proteins including PGC-1α, SIRT-1, Fox1a, eNOS, and Fox3 in aging after cardiorespiratory fitness increase by exercise or resveratrol, and combining exercise and resveratrol. Autophagy signaling pathways include Atg 7, Bechin 1, and LCS-11 and inflammation-related proteins, TNFα, and NF-KB. The failure of cardiorespiratory fitness combining exercise and resveratrol to activate PGC-1α, SIRT-1, and Fox1a in certain models could explain the inability of resveratrol to regulate exercise endurance in the report [24]. The effects of cardiorespiratory fitness increases by exercise and resveratrol intake in cardiomyocytes were determined to be PGC1α and SIRT1-dependent, suggesting that the effector molecule responsible for improved mitochondrial function with resveratrol treatment is PGC1α, regardless of how it is activated. Despite this rapid clearance, studies in animals and in humans have shown that oral administration of resveratrol protected against the development of various cardiovascular and metabolic diseases. Increased expression/activity of endothelial NO synthase (eNOS) in response to resveratrol treatment is a critical factor in increasing NO levels. These effects of cardiorespiratory fitness increased by exercise training on the resveratrol-induced increase of NO bioavailability involved higher expression/activity of eNOS [13]. MEK1/2 and ERK1/2 regulated left ventricular hypertrophy interaction cardiorespiratory fitness with NFATc3 and calcineurin. NFATc3 and calcineurin control left ventricular pathologic hypertrophy resulting in MEK1/2 and ERK1/2 regulation of physiologic left ventricular hypertrophy in different cardiorespiratory fitness. Thus, cardiorespiratory fitness is increased by exercise training, resveratrol intake, and a combined exercise and resveratrol induce physiologic and pathologic transition. As we know, MEK1/2 and ERK1/2 identified left ventricular physiologic hypertrophy, however, NFATc3 and calcineurin are identified as left ventricular pathologic hypertrophy [25]. Some reports show that not find ERK1/2 and NFATc3 were binding together. Thus, we could know exercise training will improve cardiorespiratory fitness with resveratrol intake, and combining exercise and resveratrol induces physiologic hypertrophy, but not pathologic hypertrophy.

6. Conclusion

In addition, the combination of high-tech advanced medical care, genomic personalization medicine, and preventive medicine will become the focus of the future development of the biotechnology industry [26]. Also adheres to the cross-domain integrated development to improve people's health and quality of life, and provides a consultant model to assist medical care. The clinic promotes personalized anti-aging programs, natural nutritional prescriptions, and preventive medical health management to awaken the body's original anti-aging self-healing power, allowing everyone to reverse the sub-healthy and healthy life. The management consultant of a comprehensive medical clinic, if the benefits are significant, will be expanded to other medical clinics in the future to achieve cross-domain integrated development.

Conflict of interest

None of the authors has conflicts of interest to declare.

Authors contributor

All authors read and approved the final manuscript.

Author details

Jia-Ping Wu[1,2]*, Zhu Xiaoning[1], Li Xiaoqing[1], Zhang Jie[1] and Zhang Qian-Cheng[1]

1 Department of Medical Technology, Shaoguan University Medical College, Shaoguan City, Guangdong Province, China, China, P.R.C.

2 Department of Nursing, Shaoguan University Medical College, Shaoguan City, Guangdong Province, China, China, P.R.C.

*Address all correspondence to: wujiaping20227050@sgu.edu.cn; wu20227050@163.com

References

[1] Li S, Fasipe B, Laher I. Potential harms of supplementation with high doses of antioxidants in athletes. Journal of Exercise Science and Fitness. 2022;**20**:269-275

[2] Pizzorno J. Strategies for protecting mitochondria from metals and chemicals. Integrated Medicine (Encinitas). 2022;**21**:8-13

[3] Papadopoulos KI, Sutheesophon W, Aw TC. Too hard to die: Exercise training mediates specific and immediate SARS-CoV-2 protection. World Journal of Virology. 2022;**11**:98-103

[4] Sheweita SA, El-Masry YM, Zaghloul TI, Mostafa SK, Elgindy NA. Preclinical studies on melanogenesis proteins using a resveratrol-nanoformula as a skin whitener. International Journal of Biological Macromolecules. 2022;**223**:870-881

[5] Song A, Cho GW, Moon C, Park I, Jang CH. Protective effect of resveratrol in an experimental model of salicylate-induced tinnitus. International Journal of Molecular Sciences. 2022;**23**:14183

[6] Kobylka P, Kucinska M, Kujawski J, Lazewski D, Wierzchowski M, Murias M. Resveratrol analogues as selective estrogen signaling pathway modulators: Structure-activity relationship. Molecules. 2022;**27**:6973

[7] Liu M, Wang C, Ren X, Gao S, Yu S, Zhou J. Remodelling metabolism for high-level resveratrol production in Yarrowia lipolytica. Bioresource Technology. 2022;**365**:128178

[8] Wolf A, Fink T, Hinkelbein J, Mertke T, Volk T, Mathes A. Resveratrol therapy improves liver function via estrogen-receptors after hemorrhagic shock in rats. PLoS One. 2022;**17**: e0275632

[9] Qureshi N, Desousa J, Siddiqui AZ, Morrison DC, Qureshi AA. Reprograming of gene expression of key inflammatory signaling pathways in human peripheral blood mononuclear cells by soybean lectin and resveratrol. International Journal of Molecular Sciences. 2022;**23**:12946

[10] Konopko A, Litwinienko G. Mutual activation of two radical trapping agents: Unusual "Win-Win Synergy" of resveratrol and TEMPO during scavenging of dpph$^{\bullet}$ radical in methanol. The Journal of Organic Chemistry. 2022;**87**:15530-15538

[11] Gherardi G, Corbioli G, Ruzza F, Rizzuto R. CoQ_{10} and resveratrol effects to ameliorate aged-related mitochondrial dysfunctions. Nutrients. 2022;**14**:4326

[12] Qin X, Luo H, Deng Y, Yao X, Zhang J, He B. Resveratrol inhibits proliferation and induces apoptosis via the Hippo/YAP pathway in human colon cancer cells. Biochemical and Biophysical Research Communications. 2022;**636**:197-204

[13] Cao X, Liao W, Xia H, Wang S, Sun G. The effect of resveratrol on blood lipid profile: A dose-response meta-analysis of randomized controlled trials. Nutrients. 2022;**14**:3755

[14] Guo S, Zhou Y, Xie X. Resveratrol inhibiting TGF/ERK signaling pathway can improve atherosclerosis: Backgrounds, mechanisms and effects. Biomedicine & Pharmacotherapy. 2022;**155**:113775

[15] Zhai L, Zhang Z, Guo L, Dong H, Yu J, Zhang G. Gefitinib-resveratrol cocrystal with optimized performance in dissolution and stability. Journal of Pharmaceutical Sciences. 2022;**111**: 3224-3231

[16] Komorowska D, Radzik T, Kalenik S, Rodacka A. Natural radiosensitizers in radiotherapy: Cancer treatment by combining ionizing radiation with resveratrol. International Journal of Molecular Sciences. 2022;**23**:10627

[17] Zeng XL, Yang XN, Liu XJ. Resveratrol attenuates cigarette smoke extract induced cellular senescence in human airway epithelial cells by regulating the miR-34a/SIRT1/NF-κB pathway. Medicine (Baltimore). 2022;**101**:e31944

[18] Agbadua OG, Kúsz N, Berkecz R, Gáti T, Tóth G, Hunyadi A. Oxidized resveratrol metabolites as potent antioxidants and xanthine oxidase inhibitors. Antioxidants (Basel). 2022;**11**:1832

[19] Wang L, Lai C, Li D, Luo Z, Liu L, Jiang Y, et al. Lecithin-polysaccharide self-assembled microspheres for resveratrol delivery. Antioxidants (Basel). 2022;**11**:1666

[20] Wang L, Shao M, Jiang W, Huang Y. Resveratrol alleviates bleomycin-induced pulmonary fibrosis by inhibiting epithelial-mesenchymal transition and down-regulating TLR4/NF-κB and TGF-β1/smad3 signalling pathways in rats. Tissue & Cell. 2022;**79**:101953

[21] Ben-Zichri S, Rajendran S, Bhunia SK, Jelinek R. Resveratrol carbon dots disrupt mitochondrial function in cancer cells. Bioconjugate Chemistry. 2022;**33**:1663-1671

[22] Brockmueller A, Mueller AL, Shayan P, Shakibaei M. β1-Integrin plays a major role in resveratrol-mediated anti-invasion effects in the CRC microenvironment. Frontiers in Pharmacology. 2022;**13**:978625

[23] Xu J, Sun L, He M, Zhang S, Gao J, Wu C, et al. Resveratrol protects against zearalenone-induced mitochondrial defects during porcine oocyte maturation via PINK1/Parkin-mediated mitophagy. Toxins (Basel). 2022;**14**:641

[24] Mendoza A, Karch J. Keeping the beat against time: Mitochondrial fitness in the aging heart. Frontiers in Aging. 2022;**3**:951417

[25] Gutlapalli SD, Kondapaneni V, Toulassi IA, Poudel S, Zeb M, Choudhari J, et al. The effects of resveratrol on telomeres and post myocardial infarction remodeling. Cureus. 2020;**12**:e11482

[26] Yang S, Sun M, Zhang X. Protective effect of resveratrol on knee osteoarthritis and its molecular mechanisms: A recent review in preclinical and clinical trials. Frontiers in Pharmacology. 2022;**13**:921003